NATURAL REMEDIES

For Common Complaints

Belinda Grant Viagas N.D., D.O., Dip.C. has been involved with healing and natural healthcare since her early twenties, when she first consulted a naturopath. She is based in London and travels widely with her teaching and workshop programme. She may be contacted c/o the publishers.

BELINDA GRANT VIAGAS

NATURAL REMEDIES

For Common Complaints

PIATKUS

To Neil Pilkington

© 1995 Belinda Grant Viagas

Published in 1995 by Judy Piatkus (Publishers) Limited
5 Windmill Street
London W1P 1HF

The moral right of the author has been asserted
A catalogue record for this book is available from the British Library

ISBN 0–7499–1443–2

Designed by Paul Saunders
Illustrations by 1-11 Line-art

Typeset by Phoenix Photosetting, Chatham
Printed by Bookcraft (Bath) Ltd

CONTENTS

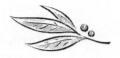

A-Z of Complaints

Diagrams

ACKNOWLEDGEMENTS

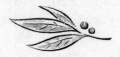

My thanks to Betty Balcombe and Simon Tapsell, who were both there for me when I needed help, and to Raymond Harris for his patience and kindness. Dick Kelly always managed to cheer me up and makes a great lunchtime companion. My mother, Nora Viagas, helped me to rediscover the sweet medicine of good companionship and laughter and provided a place for me to be inspired and loved.

INTRODUCTION

Health is not simply a physical matter. It is about finding happiness, spiritual fulfilment and peace of mind, along with physical ease. Good health means feeling good about ourselves and the things we do, every bit as much as it is concerned with how we look after our bodies. This book is a guide to simple and effective natural remedies that can be used to enhance overall health through treating a wide variety of health concerns.

Natural remedies work by restoring balance and harmony to the person. Unlike pharmaceutical drugs and chemical replicas of natural substances they do not upset the system or cause negative side effects. The remedies work specifically to strengthen the individual on a physical level and also heal by deepening our connection with the natural world.

It is when we feel separate and isolated from nature that many health concerns begin. This doesn't mean that we need to return to pre-industrialised times (although sometimes I wonder . . .), but rather that we need to wake up to the fact that however much we try to insulate ourselves in concrete forests, surrounded by technnological artefacts, we are in fact a part of nature and that aspect of ourselves needs to be acknowledged. This is the aspect of ourselves that responds to a beautiful sunset, that feels uplifted by a walk in a wood or by the way that sunlight seems to play upon a body of water. If ever we doubt the connection between mind and body we need only to witness our inner feelings when faced with a beautiful landscape on a spring day or when walking barefoot along a beach as the warm sand shifts and envelops each new step. Experiencing this feeling of connection with nature influences us not just physically; it also improves our emotional outlook and our general humour.

It is of little surprise if we become unwell through distancing ourselves from these natural experiences. It is almost as if a part of us pines and starts to wither if deprived of such beauty on a day-to-day level. It is an old saying that 'the eyes are the window to the soul', and it can indeed feel as though we are being touched in a place deep within ourselves by the sight of a beautiful scene in nature, or by the sunlight warmly reaching into us after a long winter.

Our lives can be lived in harmony with the natural world or in competition with it. We all need to make that choice and then live it. We can choose on a daily level to fight nature in its constant work towards balance, or we may choose to assist it, giving help and encouragement, and gentle support when needed. The plants, stones, minerals and elements of nature that are all around us will assist us both practically and through what they may represent for us. If we accept our own basic goodness and that we are constantly moving towards total health on every level of our being then the obvious thing to do is to enhance that process. To gently support and nurture our own growth is the natural way.

Treating oneself is an empowering act, and taking responsibility for our health and healing is an important step in our individual growth. There is a tendency in our society to make the individual feel ignorant of, and disenfranchised from their own body. Reclaiming our ability to respond to our own needs is a vital piece of personal integration. The suggestion is not that we all need to undertake a healer's training course of some kind, rather that we remember that we always have a choice in our pursuit of total health. For some that may mean having their health diagnosed by a practitioner and then deciding on their own treatment plan. Others may choose to make more time for their healthcare and give a greater priority to this aspect of their lives.

The body responds remarkably well to being listened to. When it is at last regarded as important enough to be heard, responded to and treated gently, and the whole person is physically, emotionally, mentally and spiritually working towards the same purpose, the outcome is an awesome thing – an express train of health and happiness shooting through any imbalance and disharmony. Taking steps to restore natural balance to the whole being is rather like aligning the tracks for the train to run along.

There is also a lot of fun to be had in responding to our body's needs in this way. Happiness is as important a part of full health as a heartbeat, and laughter is strong medicine. Even the bitterest herb can seem like a friend when we know it is just what the body needs. It is worth remembering, too, that all the salad you can eat won't make you better if you resent every mouthful!

Some of the suggestions in this book are for releasing pent-up energies or exploring creativity. These lie alongside recommendations about specific foods to eat or exercises to begin, making a wonderful medley of natural measures to support full health.

I find natural healthcare very exciting because of the opportunities it offers for personal discovery and self-responsibility. That nature contains all we need for continued good health fills me with a sense of wonder and fuels my enthusiasm for experiencing a range of different ways to meet the body's needs.

I find it tremendously exciting that walking on grass wet with early-morning dew or sitting by a waterfall should be as important a therapeutic measure as taking a herb tea three times a day or avoiding caffeine. When it comes to more serious complaints, there is a quiet joy to be found in the fact that there is always a range of natural answers to any difficulty. Embracing natural healthcare gives us permission to experience that childlike sense of wonder in the world and to marvel at its workings while also offering us a practical way of looking after ourselves.

How to
Use This Book

All the remedies in this book are natural. This means that they incorporate elements of nature and are not invasive. I have chosen an assortment of physical measures, including diet and the use of plants, stones and the elements, and combined them with aspects of a number of different healing systems.

Many of these remedies are steeped in country lore and known as witches' or old wives' tales. Modern science is slowly catching up and confirming their validity – many pharmaceutical drugs are essentially chemical copies of the active principles to be found in plants and foods. The benefits of using substances in their natural form are that there are no side effects, they are easily accessible, and can be quickly applied.

All the remedies described here have a positive effect. They come from a variety of sources, many of which are available in and around the home, and there is no need for extensive preparation. Foods, plants and natural energies make available to us almost everything we need for continued good health, and they are there for us when we need them.

Most of the entries in this book list a number of different treatment options and you may well find that some work better for you than others. This may change according to the seasons and your own internal timing. Women may also find that they respond more sensitively to any remedy at different points in their cycle. As with all remedies, extra care needs to be taken during pregnancy, and in my opinion this is a time when nothing other than food should be taken without the advice and monitoring of a natural healthcare practitioner.

If you use these remedies as recommended they should not cause any side effects or other problems. If you do not feel better after using any remedy, however, or if there is no change in your symptoms after three days, it may be time to contact your naturopath or natural healthcare practitioner. This may also be true if you find yourself consulting this book a lot or if the same symptoms return often – it may be that you need more personalised advice that is tailored to suit your own constitution and needs.

Psychics and other people who are sensitive to remedies will find that the recommendations are conservative and should suit them. If worried, though, cut the doses in half and reduce their frequency.

TYPES OF REMEDIES

Here is some useful information on the different types of remedies you will find in the A–Z of Common Complaints.

ESSENTIAL OILS

These are concentrated essences that have been extracted from plants. They can be used in a number of ways but they should not be applied to the skin without first being diluted in a carrier or base oil or, on occasion, water. They are extremely potent and two or three drops will go a long way. Some shops sell what they call essential oils, yet if you read the label you will see that they are already heavily diluted. Often the price will be a good indicator, but if you are at all unsure then check the label.

Essential oils are most often used by aromatherapists, who mix them with a carrier or base oil and treat through massage. This is one of the ways that the essential oils may be used at home, and they may also be added to the bath, used as a room scent by being placed in a bowl of warm water or added to an oil burner, or used in compresses, steam inhalations and other therapeutic applications.

Unless otherwise suggested, two drops of essential oil is sufficient to add to any amount of water, from a bowl for infusion to a whole bath. Two to four drops will be sufficient to add to any amount of a carrier oil from 1 tablespoon to 1 cupful. You can then increase the amounts proportionately.

Pure unroasted sesame oil is one of the best oils to use as a carrier. Do not use the ripened, dark-brown sesame oil that is so good for cooking; rather the pale, beautifully aromatic oil that can be found in some health-food shops or from specialist suppliers.

Olive oil also makes a lovely base oil. It is especially useful for small areas or patches of hard skin which will benefit from this thick, deeply scented oil. Other oils may be used too, and it is worth experimenting to see which one you feel most happy with. Those to try include almond and apricot kernel oils, which are both very good for dry skin and for facial use, wheat-germ oil, which is high in vitamin E, and the readily available soya oil. Small bottles of all these oils may be obtained from your health-food shop or from specialist suppliers.

The essential oil of clary sage has marked mood-enhancing qualities and for this reason needs to be used cautiously. I strongly advise that you don't drink alcohol, operate machinery or drive a car within hours of exposure to the oil. In fact, this oil is often best used close to bedtime for its excellent effect on dreams.

HERBS

Herbs are plants, and they can be used like vegetables in many instances, added to salads, juiced or made into soups. They may also be dried and made into teas, added to baths or used in other ways. Herbs may also be taken as tinctures – this is when the active property of the herb is extracted through alcohol, which is then taken in a presciption of so many drops a day. This makes a strong dose of the herb easily accessible, although it may preclude its use by some people. I often recommend the tincture echinacea because of its excellent ability to stimulate the immune system, although the juice of the fresh herb can be taken instead, while a tea made from the dried leaves is less potent.

Many different ways of using herbs are suggested in this book. Wherever possible it is best to use fresh herbs, and dried herbs can often be substituted if the quantities are adjusted. For teas and all other recipes, substitute half the amount of dried herbs for fresh, e.g. when 2 tablespoons of the fresh herb is suggested, 1 tablespoon of the dried herb may be substituted.

How to Make Compresses

THESE are often used to speed the healing of wounds and other soft-tissue injuries and can be used either hot or cold.

To make a simple compress, wet a piece of cotton fabric under the appropriate hot or cold tap and wring it out until it is no longer dripping. Apply it to the affected area and either hold it in place by hand or keep it there by some form of wrapping (a dry, freshly laundered tea-towel is ideal). A hot compress may be wrapped up with a hot-water bottle for prolonged effect.

To make a herbal compress, soak the cotton fabric in a herbal infusion, tincture or other extract. For a hot compress, heat the liquid gently without letting it boil. Herbal compresses are most often left in place until they have dried. Essential oils may be added to a compress by diluting a few drops in a bowl of water and immersing the fabric in it.

How to Make a Poultice

THIS has a similar action to a compress, but the whole vegetable or herb is applied and it tends to have a more drawing effect. They are most often applied hot but the application of cold, freshly picked leaves is also sometimes called a poultice. Potatoes and aloe are both examples of good healing poultices that can be applied raw for best effect.

For a hot poultice, put the substance in a non-aluminium saucepan with a few drops of water and heat gently until boiling. Place the mush on a strip of gauze or other piece of thin cotton fabric and apply to the affected area, which has first been treated with either a drop of pure unroasted sesame oil or a dab of calendula cream to ensure the poultice will not burn or stick to the skin. Larger, more fibrous leaves such as cabbage may need to have any large spines crushed before application. Either hold the poultice in place by hand or wrap it with a bandage or clean dry tea-towel.

A bread poultice is made by adding boiling water to a bowl containing crustless bread. This is then wrung out in a strip of cotton fabric or a freshly laundered tea-towel until all excess moisture is removed. A bread poultice is one of the most effective ways of drawing toxins from the body and can be used for everything from splinters to wound infections.

TISSUE SALTS

There is a range of 12 mineral or tissue salts in a gentle form that can be easily and quickly absorbed by the body. They were devised over a century ago by a Dr Schuessler, who isolated 12 minerals which he felt were vital to healthy cell function. Today these are known by their abbreviated Latin names, e.g. Ferr. Phos. (iron phosphate) and Kali. Mur. (potassium chloride).

Each pot of tissue salts contains hundreds of tiny, slightly sweet-tasting pills, which will dissolve on the tongue and enter the bloodstream almost instantly. Take as directed on the pot in either the acute or chronic dose. Acute conditions are those that are short-lived and appear suddenly – in these cases the tissue salts can show effects within hours. There is a different dose for chronic, or long-standing, conditions, and it may take longer to see a change if difficulties have been present for some time.

The pills are generally taken two to a dose by decanting them into the lid of the pot and then popping them straight from the lid into the mouth. This way they do not need to be handled. New Era, one of the two companies that now market tissue salts, also sells combinations of salts as remedies for specific conditions, and these are called Combinations A–S. Tissue salts can be obtained from most health-food shops and a growing number of chemists.

DR BACH'S FLOWER REMEDIES

These are the distilled essences of a variety of flowers and they work very well on an emotional level as well as on the body systems. Dr Bach, who originated these remedies, divided them into treatments for seven different general types – those for treating over-sensitivity; fear; uncertainty or indecision; lack of interest in the present; despondency and despair; over-concern for the welfare of others; and loneliness. Perhaps the best-known is the combination called Rescue Remedy, which is helpful in all those situations where we may feel in need of rescuing – from shock to exam nerves and visits to the dentist.

The remedies are available in 10ml and 20ml dropper bottles and the usual dosage is two to three drops in a small glass of water that is sipped slowly. This can be repeated several times daily and especially on rising and before bed. The drops may also be taken directly on the tongue. They all contain alcohol so some people may prefer to apply the drops to the pulse spots in their wrists and neck rather than drink them. Rescue Remedy may also be bought as a lanolin-free cream for ease of application.

SUPPLEMENTS

In an ideal world we would be able to obtain all the nutrients we need from the food we eat. Bearing in mind the questionable nutritional quality of our foods and the additional stresses that are placed on our bodies, deficiencies do occur and this can make supplementation essential. Specific health concerns can also increase the need for individual vitamins or minerals.

As a general rule, vitamins and minerals can be divided into two types – natural and synthetic. The natural ones are obviously the best ones to take. They will most often be packaged without the preservatives, colourings, flavourings and sugars that may be present with synthetic, chemical copies. As with so many things today, reading the label carefully is the only way to ensure that you buy what you are looking for.

Individual vitamins are often recommended in this book as part of a remedy, but taking an all-round multi-vitamin and mineral supplement during the autumn can really help reduce the number of minor complaints throughout the winter months.

Vitamin C is particularly interesting. It has a protective effect and can help fight off a cold by strengthening the immune system. Where indicated, take 1g up to three times a day, with food.

Large amounts can be taken because the body has a very simple way of protecting against overdose: when enough vitamin C is present in your system you will get mild diarrhoea within two hours of your last dose. Stop at this stage, don't take any for half a day, and then reduce the dose to twice daily, or even once. It is important to reduce your intake gradually because the body can react with scurvy-like symptoms if a high-level dosage is suddenly abandoned.

Vitamin C can be hard if taken on an empty stomach, so try to buy a buffered or 'gentle' supplement and, if possible, one that includes bioflavonoids. These occur in nature whenever the vitamin is present and they help with its absorption. If you cannot find such a combination C supplement, eat a piece of fruit minutes before you take it.

HOMOEOPATHIC ARNICA

Homoeopathy is an entirely separate system of medicine with its own laws, methods and rationales. It is not essentially an aspect of natural healthcare. However, one particular remedy, Arnica, is so useful that I have included it here. Arnica relieves the shock of injury, aids the reabsorption of bruises and stimulates circulation. It can be taken for as long as the injury is troublesome and for one week after full use is regained, switching to the chronic dose once symptoms have ceased or mobility has returned. It is now marketed by two companies and can be found in all health-food shops and many pharmacies. The dosage varies slightly, so follow the instructions on the pack. The terms acute and chronic refer to the incidence of the complaint that you are taking the remedy for. Acute means it has only recently happened, and you have just begun taking the remedy. Chronic means that it is an ongoing or old complaint, and/or that you have been taking the remedy for some time.

Do not consume any food or drink 20 minutes before or after taking arnica. Any strong flavours, such as peppermint, coffee and eucalyptus, can have the effect of nullifying homoeopathic remedies so it is best to avoid them. Should you wish to antidote the remedy for some reason, then several cups of strong coffee would certainly do that.

WHERE TO OBTAIN THE REMEDIES

Any remedies that are not already in your kitchen cupboard, or possibly in your garden, can be obtained from health-food shops and from a growing number of chemists. Some specialist suppliers are listed on pages 145–51, and a good health-food shop will put you in touch with local suppliers if they cannot help you themselves.

Just because you buy something in a health-food shop, however, is no guarantee of its goodness, so do check the labels carefully. Some companies try to market goods as natural or pure even though they contain sugars, colourings, preservatives and other additives – the most outrageous example I have ever seen of this is a certain brand of Vitamin C tablet that contains sugar, synthetic orange flavouring, orange food colouring and a preservative, and all of these in greater amounts than the vitamin itself!

FINDING A PRACTITIONER

Anaturopath is rather like a natural GP – a specialist in general healthcare who can treat people for a host of health concerns and who uses a range of natural means and resources. Central to the naturopathic philosophy is the fact that 'only Nature heals', and individual participation in all aspects of healing is central to any recovery. This means that the emphasis is always on finding ways for patients to help themselves rather than just giving them a pill or a potion to take.

It is important to be clear about what natural healthcare practitioners can offer. Beside naturopaths, there is a range of specialists offering different treatment options. Some practitioners, such as massage therapists or nutritionists, work specifically with one aspect of healthcare, while others, such as homoeopaths or herbalists, work with just one system. Both homoeopaths and herbalists will often have some experience of other ways of treating, such as giving nutritional advice, and should be capable of acting as general healthcare practitioners, as would anyone trained in Ayuravedic medicine, Shamanism or Traditional Chinese Medicine, for instance.

Naturopathy has such a wide-ranging approach that the richness of treatment options is limited only by the practitioner – no two naturopaths work in exactly the same way although they all share a similar philosophy.

There are professional bodies and associations for most forms of healthcare and these will be able to tell you which practitioners in your area have attended a recognised training course and successfully completed some form of examination. Very often the best form of recommendation is from someone you know who has been successfully treated by a particular practitioner. The most important thing is to choose someone you feel you can trust and can talk to.

OSTEOPATHY AND OTHER THERAPIES

Osteopathy, an important aspect of naturopathy, is a way of directly addressing structural difficulties and influencing the rest of the body. Nowadays some osteopaths are specialists in their own right, and no longer learn these skills as part of the naturopathic philosophy. All osteopaths, however, view the body in a similar way and will treat people with a range of complaints from back pain to joint problems.

Osteopaths use a variety of techniques to make a diagnosis, including palpation (touch) and observing the way that the body moves. Once satisfied that they know the nature of the difficulty, they are likely to use manipulation to restore function to the area. A naturopathically trained osteopath is more likely to suggest exercises and other measures to support the treatment and continue the good work.

Chiropractors also work with the body but use X-rays for diagnosis and tend to employ a more direct, thrusting style of manipulation. This means that chiropractic appointments may be completed in a shorter time than osteopathic ones.

Cranial osteopaths are usually osteopaths who have studied cranial work on a postgraduate course. This treats the whole body through diagnosing, analysing and then treating any imbalances or malpositioning in the bones of the skull.

Cranio-sacral therapists work in a slightly more subtle way and place greater importance on the fluid balances of the body. They often have no osteopathic training but the similarities between the two therapies can be enormous, because there is such a crossover of ideas and methods. Neither therapy should be at all invasive or disturbing; rather they are profoundly effective methods for treating the whole body and achieving dramatic structural changes in the gentlest of ways. A growing number of practitioners draw on both sets of skills and call themselves cranial therapists or workers.

HOW TO BOOST
YOUR HEALTH

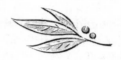

Naturopathy, or natural healthcare, is about working with the body, interpreting its needs and providing support in straightforward, non-invasive ways. All of the measures in this section will help the body by making its work easier or by boosting energy levels directly. Any or all of them may be included in your everyday routine for a healthful, stimulating energy boost while others can give you a filip when tiredness and fatigue begin to accrue.

Other supportive measures that can be found in this book include:

Dry massage – see **Abscesses**
Toning – see **Aches**
Groaning – see **Arthritis**
Circular breathing – see **Asthma**
Air baths – see **Body Odour**
Stone breathing – see **Fainting**
Foot wrap – see **Fever**
Sitz bath – see **Haemorrhoids**
Salt glow – see **Halitosis**
Humming – see **Hayfever**
Cold-water paddling – see **Poor Circulation**
Castor oil pack – see **Psoriasis**
Steam inhalations – see **Sinus Complaints**
Neck wrap – see **Tonsillitis**
Oatmeal bath – see **Eczema**
Fenugreek pick-me-up – see **Fatigue**

BODY PACK

This is a great measure for staving off colds and coughs, and can be undertaken at the first sign of flu. A body pack is a wonderful way to reduce a mild fever, and will also help ease muscle soreness.

For a body pack you will need a cotton vest, cotton T-shirt, cotton sweatshirt and a thick, natural-fibre jumper.

Line up the T-shirt, sweatshirt and jumper on a radiator and soak the vest under the cold tap until it is completely wet and as cold as possible. Wring it out until it is no longer dripping. Now, take your courage in both hands, and put on the vest (don't wear anything underneath). Quickly put on the T-shirt, sweatshirt and jumper, then go to bed wrapped up in a duvet or blankets.

You should start to feel warmer quite quickly – the cold shock lasts only for a moment – and should feel very warm and cosy before too long. There is a wonderful, secure feeling to be found in being wrapped up in this way, and drifting off to sleep is very easy. Sometimes people wake up because they have become too hot, but most usually sleep right through the night. If you wake up in the night and the vest is completely dry, then you can unpack yourself. It is not usually worth the effort, however, and is best left till morning. Then you'll need a shower, and you should find that the symptoms have dramatically improved. Packing greatly enhances elimination through the skin, taking some of the pressure off the mucous membranes, and also increases the core temperature (by raising the peripheral and subsequently the central circulation). Adults can repeat the pack twice in three days, although children under seven years old should not be packed without the monitoring of a practitioner.

If there is somebody to help you, the pack can be made up in a different way. You will need one double or two single blankets, two towels and two pieces of cotton fabric, about the size of a tea towel. If not all these items are available, a large towel, a duvet or bedcover and two freshly laundered tea-towels will be fine.

Lay the blanket(s) or duvet on the bed and the towel(s) on

top of then. Lie down on top to check where you will need to place the first wet tea-towel. You want it to cover your back but not to come too low down or to stick up out of the wrapping. When you are ready, the wrapping needs to be done quickly: you lie on one of the wet tea-towels and place the other one over your chest, and then your helper wraps you up snugly by overlapping the wrappings and tucking you up.

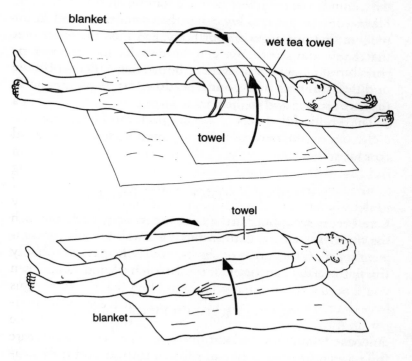

It is worth having a rehearsal with dry tea towels to ensure that you can be wrapped up quickly and that you get everything in the right place. Your shoulders need to be covered, but few things are more irritating than finding the blankets up around your nose. You will also need to decide where to do this. If the blankets wrap around your whole body, use the bed where you intend to sleep; if the width of the blankets is such that your legs are still free you will be able to wrap up on the floor, but bear in mind that you will not want to have to travel far, and movement will be very restricted once you are packed.

Although this is a lengthy explanation, the pack takes just seconds to complete, and the moments spent on a 'dry run' can make a big difference to your comfort through the night.

Arrange the towel(s) over the blanket(s) or duvet on the bed. Wet the tea-towels or pieces of cotton with very cold water, then wring out until no longer dripping. Put one on the centre of the towel. Lie down on the wet fabric and immediately place the second wet tea-towel or piece of cotton on your chest. Have your helper quickly wrap the towel(s) around you – tucking first one around your body, and then the other over that. Keep your arms above your head so that they form a tight parcel around your chest. Repeat the packing with the blankets or duvet, this time with your arms down by your side so that they are encased within the final wrap.

The wonderful effects of a body pack can be felt immediately, and by the next morning symptoms should have eased considerably.

CHEST AND OTHER PACKS

Chest packs are applied in the same way as body packs but only the chest is covered with the damp tea-towel and only the torso is wrapped. Other areas of the body may be packed too, and this is especially beneficial for the throat, neck and abdomen.

MUSTARD FOOT BATH

Add one teaspoon of mustard powder to a bowl or footbath full of water that is as hot as you can tolerate and then steep your feet in the water until it cools down. If you have a congested head or sinuses, place a piece of cold, wet cloth (a tea-towel is ideal) on the back of your neck while using the footbath.

This stimulates elimination through the skin, relieving the pressure on the mucous membranes, and also stimulates the circulation, resulting in a much warmer feeling. On its own it may well be sufficient to clear the nasal passages, but the cold compress on the back of the neck should also speed any resolution within the head and clear it completely.

Mustard foot baths can be taken twice a day if necessary, but should be avoided if there are any skin complaints such as eczema or urticaria. Children under seven years old should not take mustard foot baths without the monitoring of a naturopath or natural healthcare practitioner.

EPSOM SALTS BATHS

This is a wonderful way to stimulate elimination through the skin, improve bowel function, increase muscle tone and relieve cramps and muscle spasms. Two such baths may be taken per week, although they are not recommended for people with high blood pressure or extensive skin complaints, or for menstruating women (it may prolong bleeding). They do, though, make an excellent aid at times when premenstrual symptoms are relieved with the beginning of bleeding.

Epsom salts are available from chemists, although it is worth noting that they often sell two sizes of pack. Because Epsom salts can also be taken internally to stimulate peristalsis (the way food is moved through the gut) and as a light laxative, you can buy them in a nicely presented 50g (2oz) box, at about three times the price of a large bag and with at least six times the packaging material.

Add 500g (1lb) of Epsom salts to a hot bath and soak in it without using any soap for about 20 minutes, keeping the bathwater as warm as you can by topping up with extra hot water.

When you get out of the bath, dress for bed, wrapping up well with pyjamas, socks, etc. to maintain the effects of the bath throughout the night. Go straight to bed well wrapped up in a quilt, or duvet or covered with blankets.

Sweat through the night – most people sleep straight through because the warmth is so comforting – and shower off the next morning.

DRY SKIN BRUSHING

This is one of the most energising and invigorating ways to stimulate the whole body and has the wonderful side effects of softer skin and greater energy levels. You can brush each day, and the best time is at the start of your bathroom routine. You can brush your whole body except for the delicate skin of the face, and it takes only a few minutes to do.

With a natural bristle brush, begin by using long strokes along the soles of each foot, progress up each leg, and cover as much as possible of the trunk, always ensuring that each brush stroke moves in the direction of the heart. (Many skin brushes come with detachable long handles which can help when trying to reach the mid back and between the shoulder blades.) Then brush each hand, up each arm, across the shoulders and down the neck. The scalp may also be brushed. Avoid any areas of irritated or broken skin and try to be as vigorous as possible – it feels surprisingly good to use more pressure rather than less.

Daily dry skin brushing stimulates the lymphatic system, improves elimination through the skin and increases the circulation. It is a wonderful way to reduce congestion within the body, and its most marked effects can quickly be seen in relation to any mucus build-up in the chest or sinuses. It is a great cold reliever, but works best if you make it part of your daily routine.

The long term benefits of regular brushing include increased elimination, reduced susceptibility to colds and so on, and an overall boost to metabolism.

SLANT BOARD EXERCISES

These are exercises that are done against gravity to help tone the abdominal muscles, but they will also help to increase circulation and improve the blood supply to the head.

You will need a board that is wide enough for you to lie on and comfortable enough for you to remain on for some time. You then need to prop it up so that it is angled at a slant. Many gym suppliers will sell you exercise benches that will do nicely but, it you want to save the expense, any piece of board will do. You do need to take care, though, that it is securely placed and that there is no risk of it falling or slipping and causing you injury. Some DIY skills may be called for in anchoring it securely to a load-bearing wall.

Once you are satisfied that the board is secure you can perform any abdominal exercises on it. It is important to note, however, that a board does not reduce the potential danger to the lower back of certain straight-leg-raising exercises. Care still needs to be taken about the number of repetitions and the amount of exercise you do at any one time.

Many people, in particular those suffering from back pain and poor circulation, find great relief from simply lying on the slant board for up to 30 minutes at a time, two or three times a day. This can also be helpful for anyone who is overweight or has varicose veins or piles.

CHI DYNAMICS

This is a simple system of exercises that focuses on strengthening the individual's Chi – their vital energy or energy resource. This is achieved through reawakening their connection with the balance and harmony that is present in the universe and, working with the breath, achieving a fluidity or sense of seamlessness with these qualities.

The exercises are easy to do, and regular practice reaps enormous benefits in feelings of well-being, as well as in helping the body relieve itself of specific symptoms. As little as five minutes each day can prove a significant investment in this wonderful system, and the good feelings experienced during this time will overflow into the rest of the day.

Each exercise may be done on its own or combined with others in the book to form a short sequence, which may then be repeated as often as desired. You will find these exercises on pages 43, 71 and 82.

POTASSIUM BROTH

Potassium has a tremendously alkalinising effect upon the system, and is important to all cell function. It plays a role in such seemingly unrelated jobs as regulating the heartbeat and helping stabilise the body's fluid balance. Although potassium is found in many fresh herbs and vegetables, mild potassium deficiencies are frequent and contribute to muscular weakness, constipation and insomnia, as well as being found in most people with arthritis.

This broth is an ideal way of increasing potassium levels, and at least one mugful may be taken each day. Take a selection of carrots, beetroot (including the tops), celery, turnips, cabbage, swede and spring greens and add an equal amount of potatoes and clean fresh potato peelings. Scrub all the vegetables well but do not peel them. Place them in a large, non-aluminium saucepan and cover with water. Boil for 3–5 minutes, then cover and leave to simmer for anything up to an hour. If desired, a large bunch of parsley may be added after the broth has boiled – this adds a useful concentration of iron, yet it can have a strong flavour so it is worth experimenting with quantities. Strain off the clear broth and drink either warm or cool. The vegetables can be discarded, as all their nutrients should now be contained in the cooking liquor.

THREE-DAY CLEANSING DIET

Begin each day with a glass of lemon water. This is easily made by squeezing some juice from an organically grown lemon into a mug, adding cold water to cover and then topping it up with hot water from the kettle.

Breakfast should be taken each day, and can comprise of a selection of fresh and dried fruit (soak dried fruit overnight), with or without some brown short-grain rice. (The addition of rice can make the meal more savoury, especially if only soaked dried fruits are eaten with it.) Otherwise, a medley of fresh and dried fruit gives an instant energy lift and provides the right nutrients to begin the day. Any fruit is suitable except plums, which are quite difficult to digest, and oranges which have a congesting effect upon the liver. Melons need to be eaten on their own, but a plate of mixed melons, such as cantaloupe, water melon, honeydew and Charentais, makes a wonderful meal where nothing else is required. Individual fruits can also be eaten as a mid-morning snack to stave off any hunger pangs.

Lunch on each day should consist of a large mixed salad of

raw vegetables, including a selection of herbs and flowers especially chosen for their nutrients and flavours, and dressed with a mixture of sesame or olive oil and lemon juice. Try to include as wide a mix of salad vegetables as possible and be sure to choose some seasonal vegetables to bring further texture and goodness to the dish. A selection of shredded swede, parsnip, carrot and cabbage makes an excellent base for a winter salad, while fresh corn kernels and grated courgette added to a dish of radicchio, lamb's lettuce, lollo rosso and cos lettuce make a wonderful basis for a summer salad.

Borage leaves, dandelion leaves, fennel, and cowslip flowers are all excellent sources of potassium and other minerals, and will have the effect of cooling the dish and improving the action of the kidneys and bladder. Any or all of these may be added to summer salads or during the late spring and autumn, when the weather is warm.

Marshmallow flowers will add magnesium, colour and their soothing qualities to the meal, while parsley, watercress and rosemary improve nutrient levels across the board, as well as imparting their own distinctive flavours to the salad.

Raw beetroot can be grated and added to salads all year round, and this has a tremendous effect upon the liver, the organ of detoxification. Sea vegetables, in all their guises, are another useful addition, since they are a good source of iodine, important for the metabolism. Garlic is a mainstay, and at least one clove (more if you are able) is to be crushed or finely chopped and added to the salad meal. During the colder winter months, add some fresh ginger root and a sprinkling of cayenne pepper as well.

The greater the mix of vegetables and herbs that you choose the wider the spectrum of nutrients and the more pleasure you will derive from the wonderful contrasting tastes. Raw vegetables can be eaten throughout the afternoon if you have any hunger pangs.

For dinner each day, make another large, raw salad but this time serve it with brown short-grain rice or millet and a selection of sprouted seeds.

It is important to drink large amounts of good water throughout the day: a minimum of 1.5 litres (2½ pints), plus lemon water in the morning and herbal teas. You can drink three cups of herbal tea each day but no honey or other sweetener is to be added. Plain hot water is a surprisingly pleasant drink that is well worth trying.

This diet may be followed for three days and can be repeated every ten days, but it is best used as an immediate response to any health difficulty. For more regular use, a personalised cleansing diet is best, perhaps with more emphasis on juicing or fasting, and this can be worked out with a naturopath.

If this three-day diet is very similar to your usual diet (a lot of people eat this way, particularly in the warm weather), then go a step further and limit your diet to all raw food or make it half raw food and half vegetable juice, introducing a juice meal and two juice snacks each day.

During the coldest weather, switching to steamed rather than raw vegetables with the rice or millet is quite acceptable. For cooked vegetables, though, limit yourself to three different types at any one meal and eat these same vegetables again at your other savoury meal on that day. Different vegetables can be chosen for each of the three days. You may also like to drink more of your water allowance hot, and if the diet is proving difficult for you, then one cup of hot potassium broth (see pages 19–20) taken every few hours may enable you to carry on for the full three days.

Try to make things as natural for your body as possible during this time by avoiding wearing synthetic fibres, eating adulterated foods, or covering the body with talc, anti-perspirants and other sprays.

It is quite normal to notice some changes while following this type of diet, and it may be of interest to chart any energy fluctuations and mood swings that occur. Changes in your sleep pattern, bowel movements, appetite, skin condition and mental clarity are all possible, and whatever symptoms prompted you to try this cure may also change and possibly even disappear. Any mild headaches or feelings of fatigue will generally be dispelled by drinking a large glass of water and taking a small amount of exercise (once around the block will often be enough). Any other complaints would be rare, and therefore best taken to your natural healthcare practitioner.

KEEPING A DIET DIARY

This is a useful way to shine a spotlight on your eating habits as well as on what you eat, and can often show surprising results – few of us are aware of the amount and pattern of our eating. It is also the best way to isolate any food allergies.

Each day record your feelings on waking, what you eat and drink and at what time, and what the weather has been. Try to note any physical changes, too: whether you notice any energy slumps or highs during the day, what happens to any symptoms you may have, and whether there are any emotional upsets or issues. Note also whether the meals you eat are cooked by you or eaten in a restaurant or at a friend's house, and whether you feel relaxed or if the meal was a business occasion or eaten on the run. All of these factors can give you information about your state of health.

Keep your diary for about six weeks to give you a true overall picture. At the end of that period, it should be easy to spot any strong connections between what and how you eat and how you feel, and a lot of other insights should appear during the course of that time.

This makes the ideal basis from which to consider following an exclusion diet (see below), which simply means eliminating problem foods and ways of eating. It will also provide valuable information for your natural healthcare practitioner should you seek professional advice. Charting your eating habits in this way may help you become more tuned in to your body's needs and its daily patterns of behaviour.

EXCLUSION DIET

If you have identified a food or food group that appears to be causing you difficulty, try eliminating it from your diet for six weeks. This should confirm if you are correct, plus you will feel better if you are not eating something that aggravates you and your immune system will get a welcome break too.

Sometimes the body exhibits an intolerance to foods because they genuinely irritate it and other times it may be that your digestive system is simply in need of a rest. At the same time as leaving suspect foods out of your diet, therefore, it is a good plan to boost your overall health and energy levels, and any of the measures in this section will help with this.

The most common foods to suspect are wheat, cow's produce, salt, refined and adulterated foods (any that are stripped of their natural goodness and contain chemical preservatives, colourings, flavourings and other additives), and stimulants such as caffeine and tannin. Yeast, sugar and citrus fruits can also cause problems, and I have seen people react to any number of foods from onions to olives. So if you suspect a food, however unlikely, trust your feelings and exclude it from your diet to see if it makes any difference.

To do this successfully you need to avoid your suspect food(s) completely, and this means paying scrupulous attention to your meals, reading labels and checking the ingredients of all ready-prepared foods or those cooked for you.

It is best not to exclude more than three foods from your diet at any one time or follow an exclusion diet for more than six weeks. If you need help with this, consult your naturopath, who should be able to advise and to monitor your progress, as well as ensure that your diet remains balanced.

Sometimes when you stop eating a certain food the symptoms will disappear within a matter of days, energy levels will increase and you will notice an overall lightening of your general mood. Even if this doesn't happen it is still worth remaining on the exclusion diet for the planned length of time, because switching around with suspect foods is quite hard on the digestive system and on the rest of the body.

If you exclude something your body has been reacting strongly to, you may have cravings for it (the most common causes of cravings are wheat, sugar and caffeine). The first three to five days of any exclusion diet may also throw up a mild headache, some irritability, or changes in sleep, appetite and bowel movements. Drinking lots of water, taking sufficient rest and relaxation, and undertaking any other supportive measures from this section of the book will help.

Once the time comes to reintroduce your suspect food or foods, don't do it just as a matter of course – if you do not feel like eating the food then don't. A good way to check is to close your eyes and imagine the food in your stomach (*not* on your tastebuds) to see how you feel. If it feels okay then go ahead, but if not then it is quite all right to remain abstemious until you are ready. If you find yourself unwilling to reintroduce a major food group and are concerned about the nutritional balance of your diet, then a naturopath or natural healthcare practitioner should be able to help.

Reintroduce the suspect food very slowly, starting with a small amount on one day, followed by a day without it, then a small amount on the next day. Follow this pattern for a week, and reintroduce only one food or food group at a time.

If you have excluded something from your diet for six weeks the body will normally respond to it immediately if at all, so if you suspect a food of causing headaches you will probably experience a mild headache within hours of eating it. If this is the case then you may need to avoid this food for a longer period, and step up your immune response (see **Allergies**). Even if you don't experience a reaction it is still wise to reintroduce the food slowly.

RELAXED BREATHING

Relaxed or diaphragmatic breathing yields a range of benefits. It tones the abdominal muscles; massages the internal organs, which improves peristalsis (the way food is moved through the gut); and it increases oxygen uptake and improves general circulation. It is also deeply relaxing and stress reducing.

It can be done sitting with a straight back, or lying down. Lying down is easier, particularly if you are overweight.

Place one hand on your upper chest (in the middle, just below your collar bone). Place the other hand flat on your navel. Take slow, full, easy breaths, and relax. If your breathing is shallow and into your chest, your upper hand will move up and down as you breathe. Ideally your breathing should be full and deep, reaching right down into your abdomen. If it is, your top hand will be almost stationary while the other hand will move up and down quite markedly. Practise for 10 minutes each day until this is the case. Once mastered, you will find that you naturally breathe this way.

A NATURAL
FIRST-AID BOX

What a magical thing it is to be able to walk into the garden and pick flowers that will add their therapeutic properties to a meal, to take plants from a windowbox for a poultice, or to pull herbs from a pot in the kitchen to make tea. For many of the natural remedies described in this book, all you need to do is a little simple gardening or take another look at the contents of your kitchen cupboards. Some remedies can be bought ready-made, and the ones I use most often are listed below.

FROM THE GARDEN

All manner of plants and herbs will grow happily in windowboxes, planters and pots as well as in the garden, so it really is a case of planting those which you feel will be most useful. The list below includes my suggestions for starting a small herbal apothecary – these plants are mostly quick and easy to grow and will reward your efforts with their beauty as well as their efficacy.

Dill	Mallow	Rose
Lavender	Plantain	Thyme
Marigold	Red Sage	Yarrow

FROM THE KITCHEN CUPBOARD

This is a list of the things I use most often, and most of them are foods that you may well have in stock anyway. Once you become accustomed to natural remedies you will probably develop your own list of items that you find most useful.

Apple cider vinegar

Bread

An ice pack or frozen peas

Organically grown lemons

Bicarbonate of soda

Epsom salts

Honey

Propolis (available from bee keepers)

READY-MADE REMEDIES

These are the remedies I keep in the house, and they seem to cover most minor problems.

Calendula cream

Echinacea tincture

Dr Bach's Rescue Remedy, plus Crab Apple, Olive and Pine Flower Remedies

Essential oils of lavender and lemongrass

Nat. Mur and Mag. Phos tissue salts

Peppermint and liquorice root teas

Vitamin C and vitamin E capsules

A–Z
of Complaints

ABSCESSES

These localised infections are often caused by bacteria entering a hair follicle or wound. They can be very painful and need to be treated with care. Hot compresses (see page 5) will help relieve the pain and inflammation and can draw out any toxic matter. A compress made with two drops of lavender oil and two drops of tea-tree (or ti-tree) oil should help disinfect the area as well as offer some relief from the pain. Replace the compress every two to three hours and, this can be kept warm by placing a hot-water bottle over the area or wrapping it repeatedly with warmed towels.

A poultice made from fresh figwort leaves is an excellent cleanser and should clear any small abscesses before they get too bad.

Echinacea tincture, if tolerated, may be taken internally to stimulate the immune system and help keep the inflammation localised, and two drops can be applied directly to the area at the beginning of treatment. When taking echinacea it is important to begin with a low dose, so start by slowly sipping 0.2ml in a small glass of water twice a day, then gradually increase the dose over about a week to 0.5ml twice a day.

Vitamin C in doses of 1g every three hours until saturation level is reached (see page 8) is an effective early step towards reducing the trouble of abscesses.

For a dental abscess, massage with chamomile granules can prove effective. These granules are available in herbal or health-food shops and are designed to help babies with teething pains, for which they work excellently. If a dental abscess is suspected, do get it checked by your dentist.

In general, careful hygiene and a good skin-care routine to improve the circulation and the sloughing-off rate of dead skin cells will help keep the skin in good condition. Never use abrasive treatments when an abscess, boil or other skin complaint is present, but overall skin brushing (see page 17) once the area is healed can help ensure that such troubles do not recur.

The skin is one of the body's basic routes of elimination

and abscesses and boils may be a sign of local difficulty or that this route is proving less than adequate. Regular skin brushing and plenty of fresh air exposure and contact are all important to keep the skin functioning at its best. You could also try giving yourself an all-over dry massage each day before you bathe. Begin by massaging your head and face with small circular movements, working strongly on the scalp and more softly on the face. Work your way over your entire body down to your toes, using long, sweeping strokes down the neck and over all the long bones and torso and full circular movements around each of the joints. Be gentle and don't rush – take as long as you need to cover every inch of your body.

ACHES

Intermittent aches and shooting pains can often be the first signs that your body is 'coming down' with something (see **Colds**). Aches that occur with good cause, such as muscle stiffness after exercise, are usually a sign that the body is suffering with an inability to process a backlog of exercise byproducts. Some gentle stretching exercise will provide the most effective help. If the problem is not isolated to one muscle, or the affected area is large, an Epsom salts bath (see page 17) and supplementation with magnesium is the best course of action. If the aches signify the beginning of an episode of ill health such as flu, an Epsom salts bath will help with the cleansing process. Individual supplementation is difficult without the monitoring of a natural healthcare practitioner but try Mag. Phos. tissue salt, taking it as directed on the label for three days.

Food allergies may also cause muscular aches and pains, and if you think this may be the problem, keeping a diet diary (see page 23) is one of the best ways to isolate any likely culprits. It is worth consulting your naturopath or natural healthcare practitioner for advice on diet and nutrition designed to suit your needs.

Specific muscle soreness can be helped by covering the area

with a warm, damp cloth to which has been added a few drops of Olbas Oil. Leave this in place for ten minutes and, if you find it helps, replace as frequently as desired. This is tremendously useful for all sorts of soft-tissue injuries, from bruising to over-tiredness.

Toning

YOU may also like to try toning. This powerful technique for moving things through and out of the body, works wonderfully with aches and pains that affect the whole body or large areas of it.

Find a quiet place in which you can be quite still. You can lie down, stand up, or sit – whichever you find most comfortable, just as long as you keep your back straight. Close your eyes and gently get in touch with the ache. Explore it and see if you can sing it – just open your mouth and imagine a sound coming from the centre of the source of the ache. Let the note be the essence of the ache and let it come out through your mouth. Sing the note for as long as your breath will allow and then repeat it again and again until no more sound wants to come. The note may well change as you go through various stages of healing the cause of the ache and its quality and timbre may vary a lot. I often find the note I am making sounds more like a groan to begin with and gradually becomes sweeter as the energy is moved out of my body.

Once you have acquired the technique, toning is a wonderfully simple way of assisting your own healing. It can be done whenever you feel like it, even without a specific complaint – just take the time to be quiet and then 'tone' or sing out the sound that your body needs to make – or perhaps even the sound that your body needs to *hear* – in order to balance itself.

ACNE

This inflammation of the sebaceous glands can add to the difficulties of adolescence but may also occur at any age. Sebum is a natural oil that lubricates the skin, and it responds to the hormonal changes that occur during puberty. Since the skin is more sensitive at this time, environmental and contact allergies can cause problems. If the skin is producing an excess of sebum and it is treated with a preparation that dries it, the body may well respond by producing more sebum to correct what it perceives to be a malfunction. Therefore an effective approach will not simply stop the effects of this imbalance but will also attend to the source of it.

A diet rich in cabbage, both raw and lightly cooked, will help improve the quality of the skin, and a regular dose of Dr Bach's Crab-Apple flower remedy will facilitate cleansing.

My favourite old-fashioned remedy is to rub the affected area with a cut garlic clove. The anti-bacterial effects of this are soon felt, and if it is done twice daily for a week, the acne should soon be responding well.

Steaming the skin over a bowl of very hot water containing a sprig of fresh rosemary and a sprig of thyme is one of the gentlest ways to clean and treat the affected area. If this is just the face than you can simply lean over the bowl with a towel over your head. If large areas of the body are involved, then a proper steam or Turkish bath may be the only way. Afterwards the skin can be toned by splashing with cold water.

Essential oils of lavender, bergamot and geranium can also be helpful, particularly if applied as part of a thin coating of wheatgerm oil. The wheatgerm oil will help minimise any scarring, while lavender is soothing and helps promote new cell growth, bergamot has an astringent action and reinforces the anti-bacterial effect of the lavender, and geranium helps balance sebum secretion. Add one drop of each of your chosen oils to one tablespoon of wheatgerm oil and stroke gently on to the affected area once a day. Great care must always be taken to ensure that essential oils are not rubbed into the eyes, but otherwise this is a soothing, healing preparation that can prove very effective.

In terms of diet, it may be helpful to reduced the amount and types of fat eaten and increase your intake of vitamins C and E, preferably by eating plenty of fresh fruit and raw or lightly steamed fresh vegetables at least once a day.

ALLERGIES

Allergies can show themselves as any of a remarkably wide range of symptoms, from sore skin, indigestion and sneezing to potentially life-threatening asthmatic responses and fevers. An allergic reaction occurs when the body does not recognise a substance as beneficial and mobilises some form of defence against it.

Some allergies, such as eczema, asthma and hayfever, tend to affect members of the same family. Others, such as lactose intolerance, appear to be the result of a genetic fault. The major factor in a number of allergies is the body's inability to cope under stress. The best approach, then, is to strengthen the constitution and enhance the body's eliminative abilities at the same time as treating specific symptoms.

With food allergies, the suspect food should be eliminated from the diet as soon as it has been identified, and this forms part of a cleansing and healing dietary approach that is common to all such episodes. As with all allergies, finding the cause is of prime importance, and keeping a diet diary (see page 23) is just one way of paying greater attention to all daily activities and then linking them to any health concerns. It is best to keep the diary for a period of about six weeks so that a true picture will have time to emerge. From that, it should be possible to pinpoint specific foods, drinks, situations, or weather conditions that seem to cause the problems.

The next step is to plan an exclusion diet (see page 23) that avoids, or makes the best of, those factors. Obviously, there is little you can do to avoid wet weather, for instance, but there are ways to minimise your negative response to the damp, like including specific warming foods and spices in your diet.

People often find that it is not just one thing that seems to cause problems but a particular combination, such as eating a lot of wheat and drinking large amounts of coffee during a particularly stressful time when the weather is damp. A naturopath or other natural healthcare practitioner can help you work out a strategy for avoiding certain foods and also give advice on areas to look at and on balancing your diet. If you are doing this on your own, it is inadvisable to follow any kind of strict exclusion diet for longer than about six weeks without professional advice.

When trying to pinpoint the cause of an allergy it's worth bearing in mind that a great many of them occur in reaction to adulterated foods and substances; reactions to things in their pure form are rare. The most common allergens – wheat, cow's dairy produce, airborne pollutants, chemicals in cleaners, soap powders and other household wares, house-dust mites and household gas – are all substances that have been adulterated in some way. The wheat that we eat today, for instance, bears little relation to the wheat eaten by our forebears. It is now a product of genetic engineering and selective farming, and is usually drowned in pesticides, fungicides, artificial fertilisers and an alarming assortment of other chemicals and processes. Little wonder that the body treats this terrible cocktail as a foreign substance.

Our lungs and the delicate lining of the mouth and nose were not designed to inhale noxious fumes on a daily basis, yet anyone living in or near a city in the 1990s inhales a greater number of pollutants than our ancestors even knew existed! The effects on general health of living in a large city have been estimated as the equivalent of smoking 20 cigarettes every day.

This can all lead to the body becoming overloaded and oversensitive. Little wonder, then, that it may exhibit an allergic response to something simple in the diet, or be unable to ride the hormonal changes of a woman's monthly cycle without complaint. Rather like the last straw that broke the camel's back, the body may just be responding to too much or too many mild irritants that have been going on for too long.

To minimise the stress on your body, choose food that is in as pure a state as possible – which usually means locally grown organic produce – and water that is clear and unpolluted. Rest and relaxation are equally important aspects of any general health-improvement plan, and time spent outdoors in an unpolluted area of nature will have a rejuvenating effect upon the whole body.

Meat eaters in particular are advised to review their diets and consider reducing the amount of meat and animal products they eat each week, particularly in view of the methods used to get this food to their tables. The way in which animals are raised for food is really disgraceful – these creatures are treated more like manufactured products, shown little care or respect and allowed no dignity. Apart from the dishonour involved in supporting such a dirty business, there is also an impact upon the consumer from the large amounts of chemicals, antibiotics and other drugs found in the flesh of these animals and the presence of all the metabolic byproducts of the severe stress and pain felt by the animals during their lifetime and on the day of their death.

Many people seem to need to eat meat, and their health can deteriorate if this protein is not available. If this is the case, there are many farms and suppliers whose animals are given good lives with plenty of exercise, fed appropriate diets, and then humanely killed. This type of produce is becoming more widely available and many supermarkets now stock it.

Specific measures, such as taking vitamin C up to saturation dose (see page 8), and eating at least five portions of organically grown fresh fruit and vegetables each day, will help boost the immune system and support all cell functions. Echinacea tincture (if tolerated) may also be taken, starting with a daily dose of 0.2ml in water and slowly increasing that to 2ml.

Vitamins A and E are both important in helping the body to fight stress. They are found in a variety of foods, including olive oil and seed oils, coconut, wheatgerm, apricots, papayas, yellow vegetables (corn, squashes, etc.), lettuce and watercress. These vitamins may also be taken as a supplement, but it is best to take them as part of a combination multi-vitamin and mineral rather than individually.

If the body is exhibiting signs of allergies these general measures will help. Allergies are really the body's cry for help, and attending to its deeper needs for cleansing and detoxification will ensure good health in the future.

See also **Eczema**, **Asthma** and **Hayfever**.

ALOPECIA

Alopecia (temporary baldness or severe hair loss) can have any number of causes and may be difficult to treat. This can be a response to physical stress – post-pregnancy hair loss is a good example of this – or to emotional or psychological stresses, and these may be harder to pinpoint.

The distress that this condition can cause can be effectively treated with Dr Bach's Rescue Remedy, an aid for all kinds of shock. This should be taken as directed on the bottle. The challenge, however, is to find the cause of the alopecia.

For mild hair loss, a full-spectrum vitamin and mineral supplement is an essential first step, as is massage of the scalp and neck. This can be done each evening and no oil is needed; simply use gentle, slow and stimulating circular movements over the entire area. Once a week, massage the scalp with a mixture of two drops each of lavender and thyme essential oils in half a small cup of equal quantities of almond and jojoba oil. Afterwards, wrap your head in a warmed towel and keep in place for as long as possible, ideally going to bed with it on and washing the oils off in the morning. These two oils are said to stimulate hair growth but I feel the effectiveness may well be due to stimulating the area through massage.

The homoeopathic remedy arnica stimulates circulation and can be taken as directed on the pot. It is also a good remedy for shock, so is an ideal support at this time. Try also taking a teaspoon of sesame seeds before breakfast every morning for a month

Hair loss is a frightening experience, particularly for women, who face many pressures within our society that are related to their appearance. An incidence of alopecia makes an ideal time to take a look at such issues and how the individual feels about them. If a physical cause can be found, then that can be treated, but this may also be an opportunity to do some repair work on an emotional or psychological level.

Sudden hair loss is a shocking and extreme way for the body to behave. A full investigation of physical and emotional well-being leading up to this event can yield a multitude of clues as to how general overall health can be improved, and it is well worth undertaking this with your naturopath or a natural healthcare practitioner if possible.

ARTHRITIS

The terms arthritis and rheumatism are often used loosely to describe a range of different complaints. Most people understand rheumatism to be a general term for muscle soreness or pain, and this is perhaps the most weather-reactive of these conditions – 'I know it's going to rain because my rheumatism is playing up' is a common prediction. Atmospheric changes can have a tremendous affect on the way we feel.

Arthritis is divided into two distinct types, osteo and rheumatoid. Osteoarthritis is the name for pain and swelling in the joints, often due to wear and tear, which means that the usual protection or cushioning that stops the bones in a joint rubbing against each other is beginning to thin. Rheumatoid arthritis is the inflammation of a number of joints and needs to be viewed quite differently. Because it is so important to differentiate between these two types of arthritis, it is recommended that you consult your naturopath or natural healthcare practitioner in order to devise a full personal treatment plan with you. In the meantime, the measures outlined here may help with both pain control and general health as well as alleviating the symptoms.

In general, comfrey ointment is a useful pain killing and healing application. One of the country names for comfrey is bone-knit and it is used widely for any bone complaints, from osteoarthritic changes to fractures. In the past, a few comfrey leaves were always added to any wound packing or splint for broken bones, as well as forming the basis of any number of ointments and salves for bone and joint changes.

The anti-inflammatory herb, devil's claw taken in tablet form as directed on the box, can provide tremendous pain relief, while yellow dock and celery seeds, mixed in equal parts to make a tea, will help cleanse the joints if taken twice a day.

Two tablets of the tissue salt Nat. Mur. taken once a day can have a positive effect in as much as it seems to help 'oil' the body generally. This is best balanced by taking the tissue salt Mag. Phos. once a week.

Both osteoarthritis and rheumatoid arthritis are often signs of frustration or congestion and any means of expression can be of great help in relieving the pain and the condition itself (see Groaning, below). The most frequently unexpressed feeling that I see in my practice is anger. This is a difficult feeling for us to express nowadays, as it is often socially unacceptable, and there are usually a number of personal embargoes against its expression. Fear is perhaps the biggest reason people don't use anger – fear of what it can do, what it will feel like, what people will think of them, and so on. To this end, any means of getting to know one's anger and finding safe ways to deal with it is a potential cure for a number of ills. Beating up cushions when there's no one around, shouting at the wall or at an empty chair, moving your whole body through a range of sharp, angry, staccato movements, are all ways that can help. My own favourite is to collect damaged and broken crockery, or buy cheap seconds, lock myself in the kitchen and throw them all at the wall or on to the floor until they break. The act of being destructive can be remarkably therapeutic.

One teaspoon of apple cider vinegar added to a glass of warm water and drunk first thing each morning is a useful way of keeping the body alkaline and reducing the build-up of toxins in the blood. This is an important aspect of both cleansing and pain control. Some specific foods have a tendency to irritate people with arthritic conditions, and they should be looked at closely to see whether any link exists between overconsumption and arthritic 'flare-ups'. The easiest way to do this is to keep a diet diary (see page 23) for the foods mentioned below and then seek assistance from a

Groaning

THE technique of groaning is a wonderful way of shifting energy out of the body. It is simple, profoundly effective and can be done almost anywhere. All you need is a place to lie down and, initially at least, to make sure you are out of earshot of other people and will not be disturbed. Once you get used to doing it you may well wish to share it with other members of the family, or colleagues or friends.

So, lie down, take a deep breath in and then groan it out. Really groan, and make it last for as long as you can. Repeat this again and again until you feel you have done enough. You will find that your groaning goes through different phases and will seem to build into a crescendo and then subside. At this point you will know you have done enough, and you may well be feeling a lot calmer, and more relaxed and energised at the same time. It is a useful technique for pain relief, but if you have also managed to shift some anger in this way then you can also feel tremendous relief and a great pride of achievement on an emotional level.

Sometimes people find that they want to bang their fists on the ground or kick their heels at the same time as they groan. If you give yourself permission to have a tantrum before you begin your groaning, then your body will go right ahead and shift the anger without you needing to feel embarrassed or shy. Whatever your body needs to do in this safe, contained way is going to be all right – you cannot hurt yourself or anybody else so just take a deep breath and go for it.

naturopath or natural healthcare practitioner in eliminating them from your diet for a short time. Foods that may cause problems include red meat, salt, red wine (and alcohol generally, although red wine is most often indicated), citrus fruits and coffee. Fish and poultry can be substituted for red meat, and this can also provide a perfect opportunity to increase the number of vegetarian meals you eat. Avoiding salt opens up the possibility of experimenting with a variety of herbs and the gentler spices in order to flavour food. Try a range of herbal teas and dandelion coffee, a great liver stimulant, in place of ordinary coffee. These measures make for a generally healthier diet anyway, so can only improve overall health.

Anyone troubled with gout, a nasty inflammation which occurs in particular joints, often the big toe joint, will find relief from avoiding foods containing purine – these are herrings, sardines, shellfish, red meat and animal organs. Eating fresh black cherries with every meal gives instant relief.

ASTHMA

This is essentially a spasm of the bronchi which leads to wheezing and breathlessness. It can be life-threatening and should not be ignored or taken lightly. It may also be aggravated, if not caused, by a spasm or an irregular wave of movements in the diaphragm. Environmental factors, airborne pollutants and being in the presence of cigarette smoke can all trigger attacks. There is often a strong family connection to be found, and asthmatic attacks most often occur in individuals who have other allergies. Asthma is strongly connected with fear, which, not surprisingly, can be generated by each attack. Dr Bach's flower remedies can help with this aspect of the condition; the range that work with fears and their effects (Rock Rose, Mimulus, Cherry Plum, Aspen and Red Chestnut) are most helpful here.

Simple things that will calm and soothe are of most benefit once an attack has begun. Even listening to soothing music and having something soft to touch will help reduce the accompanying anxiety.

Spinal manipulation can help enormously both with managing asthma and during an episode, while cranial osteopathy is most effective in working directly with any problems involving the diaphragm. (Consult an osteopath, cranio-sacral therapist or chiropractor.) Massage can also help, particularly by working along the small and important muscles that lie between the ribs. A professional massage therapist may well be able to show you how best to use this on your own.

Roman chamomile and clary sage are useful essential oils to use, in dilution, for massage, and may also be added to an oil burner or diffuser. Care must be taken not to drive or operate machinery immediately after using clary sage. To massage the torso, add two drops of the essential oil to a small cup of carrier oil.

Diet plays an important role in ensuring that liver and bowel congestion do not aggravate asthma sufferers, and regularly undertaking a three-day cleansing diet (see page 20), as well as reducing your intake of mucus-forming foods such as wheat and dairy products, should be beneficial. A liver compress (see page 5) made of Swedish bitters and applied overnight once a week will support the liver in keeping the system running smoothly, while onions are a valuable addition to the diet. They contain a substance called diphenyl thiosulphate, often used in asthma medications.

All exercises that will improve breathing have a beneficial effect; often people need help in learning the proper way to breathe. Correct diaphragmatic breathing (see page 25) can help lessen or abort attacks, and once again a naturopath, osteopath or chiropractor will be able to advise. For young children, breathing exercises can be made into games, such as blowing up balloons, blowing out candles (especially the relighting ones), and even seeing who can spit cherry stones the furthest. Adults need to be encouraged to loosen up a bit and enjoy their breathing exercises so that they will do them regularly.

CIRCULAR BREATHING

Circular breathing is a Chi dynamics exercise which has many beneficial effects. Stand outside if the weather is kind enough, or near an open window, with your knees 'soft' or very slightly bent and your arms resting loosely by your sides. Slowly breathe in as you raise your hands out to your sides and then up over your head where they meet. Hold for just a second. Breathe out as you slowly bring your hands down in a line along the centre of the front of your body till they reach your pelvis. Pause for just a second, then breathe in, open the arms, and repeat, keeping the exercise going for as long as possible. The breathing is described as circular because it is almost continuous, and the arms move around making a large, complete circle in the air (which is bisected by the body). As well as improving the quality of the breathing this exercise also encourages calm and harmony and has a sweet, meditative feel to it.

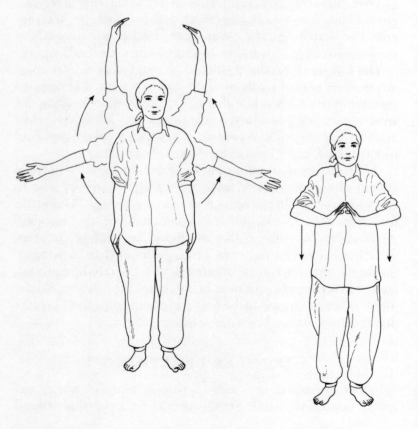

Nightly chest packs (see page 16) can be very calming and helpful for people who regularly have asthma attacks. Make sure that the pack is not fitted too tightly, to avoid feeling trapped or confined. Finally, if tolerated, ten drops of asthma weed (*Euphorbia pilulifera*) tincture taken in water twice daily can have very positive results.

ATHLETE'S FOOT

This condition is caused by a fungus overgrowth (similar to thrush) which can result in intense irritation and lead to areas of broken, bleeding skin, creating access for other bacteria. It is most often to be found between the smaller toes but may also spread to other areas of the foot. Although it is usually contained as itchy patches of dry, flaky skin there may also be episodes of abrasion and subsequent minor bleeding – mainly caused by scratching to relieve the itch.

The fungus thrives in warm, moist conditions, so feet that are trapped within socks or stockings and shoes for most of the day provide the perfect home. The gaps between the smaller toes are frequently overlooked when drying the feet, and subseqently placing them in the air-free confines of footwear is rather like putting them in a grow-bag.

Of course, most of us wear footwear, and not all of us have athlete's foot, so individual predisposition also plays a part. Changes in diet and foot hygiene can make a significant difference to the incidence and severity of this condition. Allowing the feet to breath regularly is good sense for all of us. Rather than putting already covered feet into slippers at the end of the working day, allowing your feet some freedom (an airing, if you like) is part of good foot hygiene. It is also important to remove your feet from your shoes whenever possible and just wiggle them about a bit at least once during the day. The best footwear is made of natural fibres that will let your skin breathe, and both shoes and socks or stockings should be changed daily.

Feet rarely receive a lot of attention from us and, particularly if we spend much of our time involved in intellectual pursuits, or are not in tune with our bodies, the appearance of a minor complaint such as athlete's foot can be a way of drawing our attention back to basics – grounding us in some way. Alternatively, if we are driving our body too hard, perhaps through expecting peak performance all the time or following a rigorous training routine, it can be a way of reminding us that we need to extend care and comfort to all parts of ourselves.

If you suffer from recurrent episodes of athlete's foot, removing sugar and yeast from the diet is a good long term protective measure. These foods should be avoided for at least three weeks and then slowly reintroduced a little at a time. Mushrooms and other fungi or mycoproteins should also be avoided. Eliminating sugar means not just the white, refined sort but also honey, sugar syrups, fruit juices and dried fruit. Fresh fruit is all right because the sugar contained within the cell walls is released very slowly into the system. To reduce the yeast content, though, the fruit should be very well washed or peeled.

Avoiding yeast (see page 74) involves reading the labels on everything, because it can be found not just in bread but also in alcoholic beverages, many buns, stock cubes, prepared meals, vegetable pâtés and spreads.

As a general precaution against athlete's foot, make certain to dry your feet carefully and gently after each washing and change footwear at least once a day. Use powdered arrowroot or cornmeal to dust the feet after washing instead of commercial talcum powders. These are better for the body, are not toxic and will not irritate the bronchi. Allow the feet long periods of freedom from footwear – giving them 'air baths'.

If the condition is dry and flaky, covering the affected area with honey provides the fungus with an alternative growth medium. Although it may seem strange to eliminate sugar from the diet and then apply it locally, this remedy is extremely effective, if a bit messy. Apply a thick coat of honey to the area and cover with a cotton sock. Thick set honey is best for this because it doesn't run so much. It is easy to apply before bed, but if possible it should also be done in the mornings so the foot will be covered in honey for extended periods of time. If you use it twice a day, positive results should be seen in about three days.

The strangest remedy, and yet tremendously effective, is urinating on the feet. (Men have an easier time of this than women, but then men are more likely to suffer with this condition.) I find that the easiest way to do this, for both sexes is when standing in the bath or shower. Simply pee on to the feet and let them dry naturally before rinsing off with warm water. If this proves difficult, you can urinate into a jug and then pour the contents over the feet while standing in the bath or while holding them over the toilet. Try to do this at least twice a day. Doing this in combination with the honey wrap ensures results within three days.

If the skin is badly broken and bleeding, add two capfuls of apple cider vinegar to a tepid foot bath and soak the feet in this at least twice a day. Dry the feet carefully, using cotton wool if necessary to get between the smaller toes. Once dry, prepare a solution of two drops of tea-tree (or ti-tree) oil in one tablespoon of water. Place in a saucer and soak it up with some cotton wool then apply to the sore spots; it may sting a little. Allow the feet to dry naturally, and spend as much time barefoot as possible. Once the skin has begun to heal, commence with the honey wrap and urine treatment.

An alternative to the vinegar bath is to mix together 25g (1oz) each of the following dried herbs: sage, red clover, agrimony and marigold or calendula, and cover with 1.2 litres (2 pints) of boiling water. Leave to infuse for five minutes, then strain the liquid into a foot bath. Top up with warm water and add a small splash of apple cider vinegar. Soak the feet until the water cools. This can be repeated each night until the condition settles.

If the condition has spread to other areas of the body it is important to consult a naturopath or natural healthcare practitioner – you may need to make more thorough dietary changes or perhaps undertake a more systemic treatment. It is also worth confirming that it is not some other form of skin complaint (see **Eczema** for example).

BACKACHE

Backache is the most common reason for making an appointment with an alternative practitioner and is the largest identi-
fiable cause of time off work. I believe that one of the major
reasons for this is that the allopathic approach to back problems is to kill the pain and recommend lots of bedrest. That's
rather like responding to a puncture by keeping your car off
the road for a few days and then getting in and driving it
again. If you do not do anything to repair the tyre – or to
realign your spine – it's usually only a matter of time before
you'll be back in the garage again!

If your backache is severe, has come on suddenly, or is the
result of lifting or moving something heavy, you need to visit
a naturopath, osteopath or chiropractor. These all specialise in
back care, although they use different approaches. If your
backache lasts for more than three days, or recurs, you also
need professional advice – and even if your backache disappears within three days, either after following the measures
below or of its own volition, it is still well worth consulting
one of these specialists.

When you first notice pain in your back, stop whatever you
are doing and, if it is at all possible, get into the rescue position. This means lying down on your back with your knees
raised so that your thighs are pointing up in the air and your
body forms a sort of Z shape. Placing a pile of cushions up
against your bottom is the easiest way to achieve this, or
putting your legs on a chair. Your shins should be lying flat in
the same plane as your back but about 25–40cm (12–18
inches) higher.

An acute dose of homeopathic arnica is the best remedy to
take straight away, along with the tissue salt Rhus. Tox. in a
chronic dose. These can be continued for three days. Dr
Bach's Rescue Remedy can also be taken (if tolerated),
although it does contain alcohol so may not be taken in the 20
minutes before or after the homoeopathic remedy.

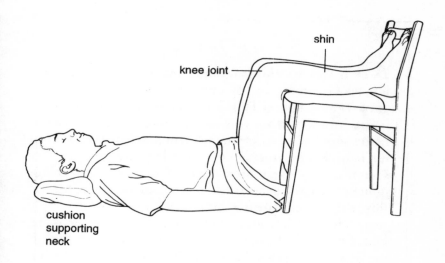

shin

knee joint

cushion
supporting
neck

Ice Pack

Iғ the pain is localised – i.e. if you can put your finger on it – an ice pack is the best immediate treatment. A packet of frozen peas works well, but anything from the freezer will do. If using ice cubes, place them in a plastic bag and then wrap them in a piece of cotton fabric, such as a clean tea-towel. Place the pack on the area and leave it there for three to five minutes. Replace it every 30 minutes for the first six hours. The pain-reducing effect kicks in very quickly and it may feel as though you no longer need to do it after a few applications, even so it is best to continue the treatment for the full six hours. (If frozen peas or other frozen food are used, make a mark on the packet – it is important to ensure that they are not eaten after having been frozen and partially defrosted several times.)

Oil of Juniper

A TRADITIONAL Mediterranean remedy for backache is to take 16 drops of oil of juniper in half a wine glass of gin every six hours. This is not an essential oil but a herbal infusion which you can buy ready made from a herbal supplier, or make yourself at home. To make oil of juniper, take one wine glass of olive oil or pure unroasted sesame or other seed oil and add 50 dried or 20 fresh juniper berries. Cover and store in a cool dark place for three to four weeks before using. As with all home-made remedies which it is hoped will benefit the person, this is best if prepared during a waxing moon (i.e. when the moon is building up to being full). The juniper helps the kidneys and the gin makes it more palatable, although home-made juniper tea can easily be made by crushing a few of the berries, covering with boiling water, and adding honey to taste, if preferred.

If an injury has been around for more than a few days it will probably respond best to warmth. Make a compress out of a piece of hot, wet cotton fabric (a freshly laundered tea-towel that has been wrung out under the hot tap is ideal), place it in the area and apply a few drops of olbas oil directly on to it. Cover with a towel and leave in place for five to ten minutes, replacing it every hour for at least three hours. Backache, particularly in the lower back, always responds well to moist heat and steam, so a warm, wet cloth is preferable to a hot-water bottle.

If movement is easy and you feel confident about your ability to raise and lower yourself, an Epsom salts bath (see page 17) is an excellent measure, likely to reduce much of the pain and also the background discomfort and accompanying muscle stiffness. If you have a heart condition, high blood pressure, eczema or are menstruating, however, Epsom salts baths should be avoided.

St John's wort oil is excellent if gently massaged into the affected area, but particular care must be taken if the back is inflamed or the skin is very red or broken.

When suffering with backache it is important to ensure that you do not make any sudden or jerky movements and that your back is well supported at all times. Getting up and down, into and out of bed, and turning round are often the hardest movements, so take plenty of time and use whatever support is available. It is much better to spend five minutes shuffling cushions around, rolling on to your side, and becoming upright in small increments, than to risk further damage to the back through speed.

Any incidence of backache can be used to advantage if it prompts a review of your exercise and postural habits. The practitioner you see will be able to advise on this and may recommend you consult an Alexander teacher, someone who specialises in movement. You may be advised to do specific exercises. These may include stretches and routines designed to strengthen the small postural muscles of the spine.

If you do not have any pain in your back at present and are not being treated for any recent injury, the following is a good overall stretching and strengthening exercise for the whole back. It can be done each day and will help keep you supple. This is not enough in itself to ensure that you will not get back trouble, but if practised regularly it will help. I find it most useful to do this exercise at the beginning of the day, on getting out of bed if possible or soon afterwards.

BACK STRETCHING AND STRENGTHENING EXERCISE

Sit upright with both feet flat on the floor. Moving very slowly, start to lower your chin down towards your chest, and at the same time bring up your arms so that you can interlock your fingers just behind the crown of your head, letting the weight of your arms encourage the stretch in your neck. Let your arms relax so that their weight is bringing your chin right down on to your chest, and let your elbows come forward to meet each other. Hold this position for a few easy breaths; you should be able to feel areas of your back and neck stretching and slowly releasing.

Slowly reverse the process, raising your arms from your head and lifting it back up so that you are looking straight in front of you. Very, very slowly let your head move slightly backwards, keeping your spine straight. Do not let your head fall backwards; rather just take it back slowly until you can feel the muscles at the front of your neck begin to tighten. At this point, jut your chin up into the air and feel the stretch down the front of your neck and at the top of your chest. Hold this for a few breaths and then slowly move your head so you are looking in front of you again.

The full stretch may take up to five minutes and can be repeated if necessary. If you do it slowly and gently, however, you will feel its effects and will not need to repeat it unless there is some specific cause during the day.

BAD BREATH

See **Halitosis**.

BLISTERS

Seasoned walkers all seem to have their own favourite herbs to help prevent and treat blisters. The most common remedy is to place a few leaves of freshly picked butterbur, plantain or marshmallow in your shoes. These herbs will all help prevent blisters occurring and can be equally effective as a treatment if they do develop.

Dancers often paint benzoin tincture or Friar's Balsam on to their toes and heels, again as much for prevention as for treatment. A few lavender leaves or flowers, or a drop or two of the essential oil, added to stockings or socks will help if less strenuous activity is planned, and these also work well when wearing in a new pair of shoes.

If blisters do occur, regular bathing in warm water to which a few drops of myrrh tincture have been added will soothe and speed healing. Blisters heal better if exposed to the air. If you do cover them, be careful not to use waterproof plasters or other airtight material – a piece of light gauze or a few leaves are best.

There seems to be a particular connection between feet and urine, because urinating on one's own feet is a remarkably speedy cure for blisters in all their phases (see **Athlete's Foot** and **Chilblains**).

BODY ODOUR

The skin acts as an elimination organ in a similar way to the kidneys and the simple act of doubling the amount of good, clean water you drink will have a positive effect on any offensive body odour. If body odour is a recurrent problem, however, your overall diet and hygiene probably need an overhaul. What comes out of the body through the pores is a good indicator of its inner condition, so skin applications are not as useful as cleansing and supporting the system as a whole. Whatever steps you can take to keep the body toxin free, unblocking the skin and supporting the kidneys will pay dividends.

Following a three-day cleansing diet (see page 20) should have an immediate effect and the diet can be repeated once a month. Make sure you eat five portions of fresh fruit and/or vegetables each day to help keep the bowels moving (see also **Constipation**). Drink at least 1.5 litres (2½ pints) of water each day and replace tea and coffee with one cup of yarrow tea per day, plus a combination of dandelion coffee and other herbal infusions. Meat eaters often achieve good results by spending a week on a vegetarian diet, since byproducts can build up in their system, particularly if the animals have not been organically reared. If this makes a big difference, you can continue eating meat as part of your regular diet, but restrict your intake to three times a week and make sure you choose animals who have been organically farmed and humanely killed.

Daily dry skin brushing (see page 17), a weekly salt glow (see **Halitosis**) and a capful of apple cider vinegar added to the bathwater should combine to support your skin function.

Contrarily enough, it is important to stop using commercial anti-perspirants and deodorants while pursuing any sort of detoxification and treatment for offensive body odour. If you follow the measures outlined here, you should find that your body responds quickly and you may decide that you no longer need to use such products on a regular basis. A light dusting of cornmeal in place of a commercial talcum powder will help maintain dryness. Wearing fresh clothes each day, made of natural fibres that allow the skin to breathe, will reduce the build-up of toxins in the skin. In very hot weather, or if working indoors for long periods, shaving off underarm hair will help too.

If profuse sweating continues to be a problem, wash your underarms and other areas where perspiration accumulates with warm water to which a capful of apple cider vinegar has been added. This can be done twice daily and very quickly settles any overfunctioning of the skin, as well as helping prevent odour.

Air Baths

Daily 'air baths' taken at the start of the day and as part of the bathroom routine, will prove tremendously helpful and will help prevent body odour. All you need to do is allow fresh air from an open window to wash over the body in much the same way as a shower. In the absence of a breeze, cover your whole body with brisk but gentle massage strokes, using both hands, and encourage the feeling of the air all over. This takes only a few minutes to do yet it feels wonderful, leaving the skin glowing and alive.

BRUISES

Bruising is the breaking of small blood vessels underneath the skin. Applying an ice pack immediately (see **Backache**) or other cold application will speed the body's removal of dead cells and other debris from the site and reduce swelling. Vitamin C taken internally in 1g doses will prompt the body's healing mechanisms and also reduce the tenderness. An acute dose of homoeopathic arnica will reduce the length of time the bruise is in evidence and is a good remedy for any type of small accident.

Crushed fresh comfrey or hyssop leaves placed directly on the bruise, or a gentle comforting massage with St John's wort oil, will reduce the discomfort and help the body.

An old-fashioned remedy is to blend a pinch of arrowroot with a little cold water and spread it on the bruise. If this is done at once, minimising the action of the air on the skin, it is said to hasten recovery dramatically.

BUNIONS

These are often painful deformities or misalignments of the big toe joint. They usually occur in both feet, if at all, although one is usually more pronounced.

The shoewear fashions of the 1950s and 1960s ('winklepickers' and stiletto heels with pointed toes) have left their legacy in the large numbers of bunions and associated problems that are troubling their wearers today. Even though such extremes of style have disappeared nowadays, the shape of the shoes we wear often bears little resemblance to the shape of our feet. You can prove this for yourself by standing on a sheet of paper and drawing around the outline of your foot, then doing the same while wearing a shoe, and compare the difference. The most notable, and outrageous, comparison is with a high-heeled shoe.

The best solution for a number of foot complaints is to wear ill-fitting shoes less often or to change your style of footwear altogether. Stockings, tights and socks that gather the toes together and increase their pointedness, thereby increasing the pressure on the bunion, also need to be avoided.

Spending as much time as possible walking around barefoot is the best therapy for bunions. The more surfaces you walk on the better: encouraging the small muscles of the foot to work well by challenging them to keep the foot together on sand, clay and other surfaces with a lot of 'give'; exciting the feet by walking in the early-morning dew on a patch of clean grass; even walking small distances on fine gravel or pebbles. Exercises that open up the toes have positive effects too; try turning over the pages of a newspaper with your toes and then progressing to a book (the pages are thicker so it is more difficult).

Gentle massage around the whole area will help too, particularly if you apply a small amount of traction and slowly rotate the toe. Otherwise encourage whatever movement is possible to begin with. To apply traction, get a firm hold on the toe and very carefully pull it a small distance straight out from the foot, imagining as you do so that a minuscule gap is appearing in the joint – just enough to allow freer movement. If the bunion is very inflamed, add a drop of chamomile or melissa essential oil to the massage oil (a small half cupful of massage oil should be sufficient). A drop of lavender, marjoram or peppermint essential oil added to the massage oil will help reduce the pain, and peppermint especially is very cooling. Regular massage sessions, perhaps for five minutes each morning and evening, will prove highly beneficial.

BURNS

If the burn is deep, covers a large area, affects the face or other sensitive areas or is the result of contact with electricity or chemicals, then seek medical attention immediately. Remember that applying fat or grease to a burn will continue to cook the skin – rather like a chip in hot oil!

Smaller burns, such as ones from cooking or friction (like a rope burn) are easily dealt with. A few drops of Dr Bach's Rescue Remedy or Rescue Remedy cream applied to the area and repeated three times at five-minute intervals soon sees off any lasting discomfort. If the burn is larger, you may need to cool it down by immersing it in cold water before any other treatment can be used. The easiest way to do this is to place the affected area under a cold tap, although soaking it in a bowl of ice cubes is a remarkably effective way of reducing the chance of blistering.

There is a magical cure for burns that arises from co-counselling philosophy, a counselling technique that allows non-professionals to work with each other. A mainstay of the teachings is that pain is caused by unexpressed feelings. Extending this to physical symptoms may seem like a leap of faith, but it makes for a truly effective cure. I would only recommend using it for small burns because you don't cool the area first, a necessity if the burn is large.

Fill a basin with hot water – test with an unburned hand that it is not too hot – and place the burned area in the basin. What usually happens is that the burned area begins to sting and after a few seconds the pain builds up to a crescendo that is enough to make you want to yowl, curse or cry. Express this pain in whatever way feels appropriate (I usually yell 'ow, ow, ow', along with a few expletives, and stamp my foot) and within seconds the burning sensation begins to subside. Keep the burn in the water until it feels absolutely fine – this usually takes only a few moments – then remove it. It will hardly be even tender to the touch – it is as though the anticipated days of soreness have concertina'd into the few seconds of pain underwater, and the burn can then be forgotten. If you remove the affected area from the water before it feels completely normal the positive effects are not so great and some mild sensitivity will remain, but it will still be nothing like the pain you might expect to feel.

If a burn is not treated and blistering occurs, never burst the blister as this can allow infection to set in. If, however, a blister bursts of its own accord, or there is scarring after a burn, the following poultice has strong rejuvenating qualities:

Mix to a paste two tablespoons of powdered comfrey root,

one teaspoon of runny honey and one teaspoon of cold pressed wheatgerm oil. Apply to the burn and cover it with a light gauze or a plantain leaf. Leave the poultice in place and add a fresh preparation to it daily. As the skin underneath heals, successive poultices will not seem to 'take' so well, or will not adhere to the skin. When this occurs, a small amount of aloe vera gel rubbed into the burn site each day will continue the healing process. I have seen some particularly good results from this, often leading to the complete removal of small areas of scar tissue.

If the burn is small, vitamin E can be applied to assist healing, but make sure the area has been thoroughly cooled first. The easiest way to apply this to a small area is by puncturing a capsule of Vitamin E intended for internal use and gently covering the burn with it. This can be repeated as often as required. Vitamin E may also be taken internally for one week or until the burn is completely healed.

Vitamin C can also be used externally to cover the site of the burn, and is usually best made into a solution with water and sprayed over the area (a new, scrupulously clean plant mister will do). Powdered Vitamin C is the most suitable for this. This can be alternated with applications of Vitamin E. Vitamin C should also be taken internally in large doses – up to 1g an hour for three hours, then three times daily for 3–5 days. This wonderful vitamin will help reduce the pain and also speed the body's own healing processes, reduce the risk of infection and help decrease any localised swelling.

If you burn your tongue or the inside of your mouth on hot food or drinks, drink a small glass of whole milk as soon as possible afterwards, holding it in your mouth for a moment or so with each swallow, and any soreness and blistering will be greatly reduced.

CHILBLAINS

Chilblains are an inflammation of the extremities, such as fingers, toes and ears, which may be caused by prolonged exposure to the cold, as well as circulatory difficulties. A dressing of freshly grated horseradish root is an extremely effective treatment, as is bathing the affected area in water in which celery has been boiled. Both can be used daily.

The best cure I know is to urinate on the chilblains at least once a day, but three times is best. The first or second urination of the day is the most potent. After this treatment the soreness subsides within a few days, and the chilblains tend to disappear altogether within a fortnight. It is a curious thing, but urinating on one's feet seems to be the best cure for all sorts of foot complaints. It is easily done if you stand in the bath or shower, or you can catch your urine in a jug and then pour it where it is needed.

Alternative treatments include painting the chilblains with raw garlic juice or nettle juice at least twice a day and drinking one cup of nettle tea each day. Good results may also be had by covering the area with a grated raw potato poultice (see page 6). This can be left in place for up to three hours or overnight and repeated as often as required.

Any measures that improve the circulation (see **Poor Circulation**) and strengthen the body will help reduce the incidence of chilblains. A diet that is high in vitamin C and fibre and low in fat, combined with good exercise and regular lymphatic support, is recommended (see the chapter on Things You Can Do to Boost Your Health).

COLD SORES

See **Herpes**.

COLDS

The common cold, conventionally regarded as the result of a virus, can also be seen as a healing crisis – a good thing! The symptoms of runny nose, sneezing and sore throat may be the body's way of eliminating toxins. There are several eliminative routes available to the body, one of which is the mucous membranes, so we get a build-up of mucus that irritates the throat, nose and sinus area, resulting in sore throat and headache. Some colds are, of course, the body's response to a virus, and here again we produce extra mucus to help defend the airways, the site of ingestion of the virus, against further attack.

Appetite is normally suppressed when we have a cold, and our tastebuds and sense of smell don't function properly, so much of the satisfaction we normally gain from eating isn't available to us. The natural thing to do here is to follow the leads that our body is giving and keep food to a minimum. The old adage 'Feed a cold and starve a fever' really means that if you feed a cold you may well have to starve a fever. Namely, if you don't help the body's simple attempts at cleansing it may just knock you out so that you have no option!

Instigating a simple cleansing diet (see page 20) at the first sign of a cold is one of the best ways of supporting your body's efforts to find its own balance. As a general rule take lots of fluids, and rely on small snacks of raw food whenever you feel hungry in the summer months, or soup or steamed vegetables and rice during the winter. You may also like to try the three-day cleansing diet on page 20.

Some people never seem to have colds while others suffer from them far too often. This raises the question of our own natural immunity. When the body is functioning well and receiving adequate rest, exercise and nutrition, the immune system can operate at its best. Often, manifesting the symptoms of a cold or similar small but debilitating health problem is the only way for a person to get the rest they need. In our busy, stress-filled lives we occasionally need the excuse of illness in order to take time out and allow ourselves the rest and relaxation that are essential for healthy living.

Environmental factors also have a part to play. If we spend too long in a dry, centrally heated atmosphere, the natural moisture of the mucous membranes can dry out, restricting our ability to repel any invading organisms. This can also have a kickback effect by encouraging the body to produce extra mucus to maintain moisture levels. One effective way to combat this is to apply a drop of pure unroasted sesame oil or a thin smear of Vaseline to each nostril.

The natural world influences our bodies, too, and it is not uncommon for perfectly healthy people to get colds each year with the change of seasons, particularly in autumn and spring. These are times when our bodies change gear and it may be that a period of rest or detoxification is needed to facilitate that change. In this case a cold is really the body's efforts at spring cleaning, and anything we do to support these efforts can have a positive, health-enhancing effect. Whenever I hear somebody say that they never get colds I worry that their internal, self-regulatory mechanisms may not be functioning at their best. It may well be that they are too out of balance to manifest a cold, and if this is the case then the immune system, and their vitality, could often do with a boost (see the chapter on How to Boost Your Health).

So it seems that, for whatever reasons, colds are a fact of life. Efforts to prevent them pay off much better than actions to relieve them, although the natural methods outlined here for cure and prevention will all enhance overall health rather than just suppress the symptoms. If you are fit and well, you are less likely to suffer minor health complaints. Ensuring a good, varied diet which allows for both treats and periods of eating simply, getting enough rest, and some form of exercise that you enjoy are the best prevention.

We can often sense the early stages of a cold, and this is the time to take lots of fluids and get plenty of rest. A relaxing evening, 1g of vitamin C and an early night may just head it off. If there are a lot of colds going around, or if you are feeling slightly under par, repeating this treatment may ensure continued good health throughout the epidemic.

If a cold does develop, switch to a simple diet with lots to drink and take 1g of Vitamin C three times a day. If this is not possible, at least avoid mucus-forming foods – all dairy products, wheat, yeast and refined sugar. Fruit can be mucus forming for some people; as a general rule, if you feel cold inside, avoid fruit. If you feel hot inside, eat fruit that has been either peeled or well washed to avoid the extra yeast present on the skin (did you know that it is yeast that gives grapes their bloom?). Take a vitamin and mineral supplement

Ginger and Coriander Drink

TAKE a piece of fresh ginger root about 5cm (2 inches) long and peel it. Chop it roughly and put it in a non-aluminium saucepan that isn't non-stick. Add about a tablespoon of coriander seeds and a couple of mugs of water and bring to the boil. Turn down the heat and simmer for 15–20 minutes, then strain and reserve the liquid. This can be sweetened to taste with honey, although it is quite delicious on its own. Drink as often as desired and at least twice a day.

Irish Cold Remedy

THIS traditional remedy hails from the west coast of Ireland where they know a thing or two about cold and damp. Although it contradicts the dietary advice to avoid dairy food, and includes sugar and alcohol, it does work remarkably well and is very tasty.

6 fresh free-range eggs
juice of 8–10 lemons
2 tablespoons brown sugar
2 large measures of brandy or whisky

Mix together the beaten eggs, lemon juice and brown sugar and then strain into a jug. Mix again and stir in the brandy or whisky. Place in a bottle and refrigerate overnight. Shake the bottle well and take a small glassful first thing in the morning.

This is enough for several days, and the alcohol will keep the mixture fresh until it is all finished. Pregnant women are advised to take great care if choosing to eat or drink anything containing uncooked eggs.

containing vitamin A and zinc. A cup of ginger and coriander drink twice a day should also help (see page 62). This helps keep you feeling warm inside, increases elimination through the skin and kidneys, taking some pressure off the mucous membranes and helps reduce the risk of 'chestiness'.

CONJUNCTIVITIS

This is an infection which causes the eye to feel sore and discharge a yellowish substance. The build-up of discharge overnight means that the eyelids are seemingly stuck together in the mornings. The rest of the day the eyes will have a tendency to appear pink and inflamed. Similar symptoms can appear as the result of an allergy or the presence of a foreign body in the eye.

Because this condition greatly affects the ability of the eye to see clearly I am always inclined to ask whether there is something in the person's life that they do not want to look at – from a desk piled with overdue paperwork to a more emotionally related incident. Sometimes the only way for us to be pulled up short and encouraged to look at something (or reminded that there is something that we're not seeing) is when the body actually does it for us.

Regular bathing of the eye with a wash made from the herb eyebright is very helpful. Add 25g (1oz) of dried eyebright to 600ml (1 pint) of water and bring to the boil. Simmer for ten minutes and allow to cool, then strain the liquid and keep in the fridge for up to 8 days. The eyebright wash can be applied to the closed eye using a cotton wool pad, or by immersion in a small eyebath.

It is important not to rub the eyes, even though they may feel irritated and hot. It is better to apply something cooling such as slices of cucumber, grated carrot or even a cold used tea bag, and lie down for ten minutes. A good remedy is to drink a cup of chamomile tea and then place the cooled teabags over your eyes. Alternatively, cotton wool soaked in rosewater is gentle and soothing.

An excellent and refreshing treat for the eyes is to sit at a table or desk with your elbows propped up and allow your head to fall forward and be supported by your hands. Completely cover your closed eyes with the palms of your hands, with the fingers coming together in the middle of your forehead up by the hair-line. Your cheekbones should appear to be resting in the heel of each hand. Make sure all the light is blotted out and then relax and enjoy the darkness and the warmth from your hands. Imagine that you are in a favourite beautiful place, such as your garden, a holiday you spent at the seaside, or somewhere you glimpsed through a train window. A place in nature is usually the most soothing, although it can be anything that will make you feel at peace. Just relax as you enjoy 'seeing' this place again. When you have gazed for a while – do not hurry this – take a few deep breaths, almost as though you know that it is time to leave and you are trying to absorb as much of the scene as you possibly can before you go. Then slowly straighten your neck, and lower your arms. When you open your eyes, blink slowly five times, then take five quick blinks and look at something in the middle distance.

This is a wonderfully refreshing and revitalising eye exercise that can be done almost anywhere. It does not need to be hurried, and if you take five to 15 minutes to do it once a day, your eyes will thank you.

Good immune system support can be encouraged during a bout of conjunctivitis by adding some supplements to the diet. Take echinacea tincture (if tolerated), 30mg beta carotene, 100mg B complex and up to 3g of vitamin C with bioflavonoids as all will help the body slough off this annoying complaint.

CONSTIPATION

Regular bowel movements are an important aspect of our everyday routine and a good indicator of our overall health. Some people have one every other day, while others experience at least two or three each day. The average seems to be one a day but the main thing is to establish a regular routine so that you know what is normal for you.

Our gut is so long that there can be a tremendous amount

of food stuck inside it for any length of time; emptying it regularly is an important safeguard against ill-health. This is particularly important for meat eaters. When the bowel is not emptied regularly this places great pressure on the body's other eliminative organs and can cause any number of symptoms of imbalance, from halitosis and offensive body odour to headaches and skin complaints.

Drinking at least 2.5 litres (4½ pints) of good, clean water and eating five portions of fresh fruit and vegetables each day are the most effective ways to ensure regular bowel health. For those with chronic constipation, a proper dietary overhaul may be the only way to get the system back in balance, and a naturopath or other natural healthcare practitioner should be consulted. For intermittent sufferers, it is important not to rely on conventional laxatives, which will irritate the bowel wall and make normal function even more difficult. Even the addition of bran to the diet will only be truly effective if at least 1.2 litres (2 pints) of extra water are drunk each day.

Taking one tablespoon of castor oil before bed will probably ensure bowel movements in the early morning but this should not be repeated more than once every six weeks. For a more frequent cleanser, take two teaspoons of ghee (liquid clarified unsalted butter) in a glass of warm milk one hour after a light supper. This may be taken up to three times a week if needed, and is best when used as a short-term fix.

My own failsafe cure is to drink several large glasses of red grape juice diluted with a quarter the amount of a fizzy water such as Perrier throughout the day. The extra liquid intake accounts for some of the effectiveness and this is by far the nicest-tasting remedy.

Slowly sipping a cup of boiled water first thing each morning may well encourage a bowel movement, more so if followed by a cup of warmed prune juice. Follow that with a breakfast of dried fruit compote containing figs, banana and dates. Put the fruit to soak the night before and gently heat it in the soaking liquid the next morning.

An excellent breakfast, or pre-breakfast drink for those with heartier appetites, is one banana blended in a liquidiser with a teaspoon of skimmed milk powder, a teaspoon of blackstrap molasses and a glass of milk. This will help ensure regular bowel movements once any longstanding difficulty has been eased.

The importance of walking cannot be overestimated in dealing with constipation. It is one of the easiest ways to keep the bowel toned and encourage peristalsis (the way food is moved through the gut). Regular walking will make a dramatic difference to any constipation sufferer, and more so if hill walking or, at a push, climbing up and down stairs can be added to the routine. This gently squeezes and encourages the abdominal muscles to stretch, as well as exercising the rest of the body. The deep breathing involved also has a positive effect as the lungs fill, pressing down on the diaphragm and gently massaging from inside all the organs involved in digestion and elimination. (See also page 25.)

CORNS AND HARD SKIN

An excellent cure for corns is to soak some bread in any type of vinegar for two days, put a piece on the corn and leave it overnight as a cold poultice (see page 6), binding it in place with a cotton handkerchief. Leave in place for three days, and on every third day soak the feet in a bowl of hot water and peel off a layer of the corn. Continue the treatment until the corn has entirely disappeared.

Areas of hard skin can be sloughed off with a pumice stone or – and this is the best excuse I know for a holiday – by walking on the beach. The combination of the salt water and the gritty abrasion of the sand makes the best foot treatment there is. Burying the feet in warm sand is a tremendously comforting, healing thing to do, and it has a host of beneficial effects on the system. At home, hot salt-water foot baths and careful rubbing with a strong towel will have a similar effect.

Any pressure points and areas of hard skin on the feet can point to postural difficulties, so a full structural assessment from a naturopath, osteopath or chiropractor is a good idea.

One of the prime causes of foot discomfort is badly fitting shoes, particularly with high heels. Even with low heels the whole weight of the body is carried on areas that were never meant to bear it exclusively and this can cause any number of difficulties. The best advice is to alternate periods of foot strain like this with time when the feet are free and unhindered.

COUGHS AND SORE THROATS

My favourite remedy for throaty coughs is to gargle with warm, strong red sage tea at least twice a day. Make the tea with three or four fresh sage leaves or one teaspoon of dried sage and a large mug of water. Let the leaves infuse for about a minute, then strain until the liquid is cool enough to gargle with. Gargle with about half the tea and then slowly sip the other half, taking care not to drink more than one cup a day. Combine this with a sage throat pack (see also **Tonsillitis**) and most problems should only last a few days.

It is advisable and extremely pleasant to drink large amounts of hot lemon and honey throughout the day; if the cough is troublesome at night, put a flask by your bed so small hot drinks can be taken as required throughout the night. To make, add a good squeeze of lemon juice and a slice of lemon to a mug of hot water, then add at least one teaspoon of honey. I favour organically grown lemons but at least make sure that you buy unwaxed ones. Another tip if the cough is troublesome at night is to raise the head of the bed by about 10cm (4 inches). This is easily achieved by placing a few telephone directories under each leg at the head end.

An old country cure is to drink the water in which cabbage has been boiled, sweetened with honey to taste. This is not as horrid as it sounds, although I prefer lemon and honey. A similar cure is to mix together equal parts of lemon juice, honey and cod liver oil and take a tablespoonful whenever the cough is troublesome. Children can take it by the teaspoonful.

I rarely recommend brands of medication but Potter's make a simply sublime cough mixture called Balm of Gilead. It is very effective and tastes wonderful, so taking it is no hardship whatever.

CRAMP

The tissue salt Mag. Phos. taken as an acute dose is the most effective remedy for muscle cramps. A regular infusion of chamomile flowers, linden flowers or fennel leaves and their seeds will help relieve muscular spasms. This can be taken up to three times a day and the liquid may also be used to soak a cotton wool pad for use as a compress (see page 5). This will help relieve any after-cramp soreness and bruising.

A common complaint about cramp is that it only appears at night time, and taking the Mag. Phos. in the evening, followed by a cup of the herbal tea before bedtime will help. Try this for three weeks out of every four for two to three months at a time, if necessary. A night application of a club moss compress will also offer great relief. Fill a small cushion cover or pillowcase with club moss and apply it to the muscle by tying it loosely with a tea-towel or similar strip of cotton fabric.

Cramps due to over-exertion will be relieved by taking an Epsom salts bath (see page 17), although this should be avoided if you suffer from high blood pressure or skin complaints or if you are menstruating. Menstrual cramps are often relieved by slowly sipping a cup of hot raspberry leaf tea or, if this cannot be taken (some people are sensitive to its high iron content), a cup of mixed lady's mantle and yarrow (see **Menstrual Difficulties**).

If the cramp is severe or occurs regularly it is probably pointing to a deep imbalance in body salts. This most often occurs as a result of continued stress and fatigue, so take a close look at your lifestyle and constitutional health (see also **Fatigue**). A naturopath or natural healthcare practitioner should be able to advise you further on building up your energy levels.

CUTS AND GRAZES

Small, thin cuts such as paper cuts will become completely pain free if you cover them straight away with Vaseline. If you have some fresh lady's mantle herb this can be roughly chopped and placed straight on to a cut for its cleansing and healing properties. Fresh plantain leaves are also good and can be used in much the same way if freshly picked and placed whole over the cut.

Grazes should be soaked and rinsed in cold water to cleanse them and encourage a fresh blood supply to the area. Adding up to 1g of soluble vitamin C to the water will help relieve the soreness and accelerate healing. A honey compress (see page 5) is the best cure and can be applied straight away, on a piece of gauze or thin cotton fabric. It is quite amazing how the skin seems to drink in the honey, and the application will need replacing up to six times in the first day, slowing down thereafter as the graze heals and the skin absorbs less and less of the honey.

The homoeopathic remedy arnica is a very effective way of dealing with any bruising that may occur, and its action in improving circulation will help ensure speedy healing.

See also **Infected Cuts, etc.** and **Bruising**.

CYSTITIS

Good hygiene is of great importance in preventing episodes of this nasty irritation, and also in ensuring that it does not become a recurrent complaint. If any bout lasts for more than three days, if there is blood in your urine, or if this is a recurrent complaint, then you would do well to consult a naturopath or natural healthcare practitioner. Repeat episodes have a tremendously draining effect on energy levels and on the immune system, so it is important to treat your whole body, not just the site of the difficulty.

Always ensure that you wipe from front to back when you use the toilet, and wash your hands afterwards. Use plain white soft toilet tissue rather than coloured, and avoid using perfumed toiletries and soaps in the genital area. Wear 100 per cent cotton underwear and, if possible, spend some time each day without wearing any. Tight-fitting panties and nylon tights are a thoroughly bad idea; try stockings instead.

Cystitis is often called the honeymoon complaint and although this rather dates it, it does pinpoint one of the main causes. Uncommon sexual activity, or rather a lot after a time of abstinence, can irritate the whole vulva just enough to cause problems. The best advice is to urinate as soon as possible after lovemaking and follow that with a long drink of water.

Contraceptive methods can also have an effect, with spermicidal creams occasionally proving aggravating. The diaphragm, with its pressure on the bladder, can be a thoroughly bad idea if cystitis has been a problem in the past. Infection can be transferred through oral sex, and what may be a minor irritation in the throat can be enough to tip the delicate balance of the vulva (and, of course, vice versa). Safer sex measures go a long way towards preventing this type of cross-infection.

As soon as there is the slightest sign of irritation, drink as much warm water as you can. This will often flush any infection right out of the system. It will be made easier if you sit in a warm bath to which has been added a small handful of sea salt. If urinating does become painful, do it in the bath and it won't feel so bad. The next most important thing to do is to keep the kidneys warm. Either prop yourself up with a hot water bottle or move your chair close to a radiator; slowly sipping a cup of hot yarrow tea will help, too.

If you are feeling strong and well, take 1g vitamin C up to saturation dose (see page 8). If you are feeling weak and a little bit trembly, limit your food intake to potassium broth (see page 19) and hot herbal teas for at least a day. When eating normally, take a broad-spectrum yeast-free multi-vitamin and mineral supplement with at least one meal each day.

If you can find fresh cranberries to juice, or pure unsweetened cranberry juice, this is an excellent toner of the whole genito-urinary system and acts as a strong cleanser. Drink as much as you like, interspersed with water. (There is a heavily marketed cranberry juice *drink* – this is high in added sugar and is not recommended for drinking as a remedy at this time.)

In all cases, slowly sip one cup of hot dead-nettle tea every day and eat some corn silk. This is the thin, silk-like string that covers heads of corn on the cob. It is usually thrown away, yet it is a good kidney and bladder cleanser. It doesn't taste of much, and eating a little of it raw each time you eat fresh corn on the cob will help tone your urinary system.

EXERCISE TO SUPPORT THE ENERGY FLOW TO THE KIDNEYS

There is an excellent Chi dynamics exercise that will encourage and support the energy flow to the kidneys. This can be done several times a day, whether or not cystitis is an acute problem. Stand up with the knees soft, or slightly bent. Lean forward slightly and push both arms out in front of the body with the hands together at about waist level (see diagram on page 72). Separate the hands and bring each arm round to the kidney at the back, by making a large sweeping movement through the air. This looks rather like a breaststroke movement from swimming, but performed at waist level. What you are doing is gathering up energy from the earth and from the air around you and scooping it back and into your kidneys. Hold your hands here for just a moment, then draw them up your sides under your armpits and reach up into the air with them. This is all done with one big inhalation.

Hold this stretch for just a moment, then bring your hands together still up in the air above your head and draw them slowly down the midline of your body as you breathe out. Keeping your hands a few inches away from your body, bring them to rest just below your navel. Pause for a moment and then repeat three times.

This is one 'layer' of the exercise. You can then repeat the whole sequence, bending the knees more and really reaching down to draw the energy up from the earth with each circular sweep of the arms. Repeat with a third 'layer', reaching down as far as possible by bending the knees. Finish the exercise with a few Chi breaths (see page 43).

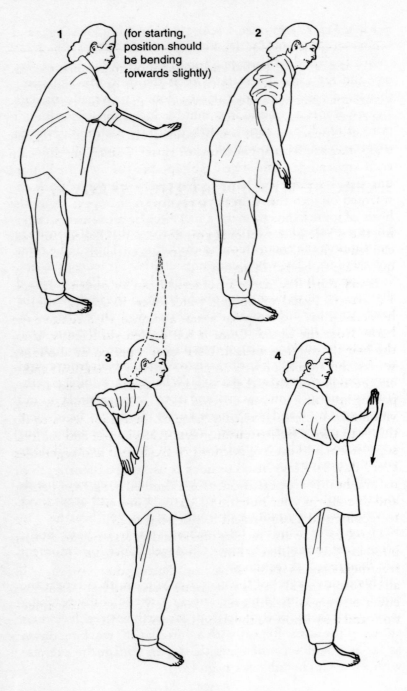

1

(for starting,
position should
be bending
forwards slightly)

2

3

4

DANDRUFF

There is a range of herbal and essential oil treatments that are all quite effective for dandruff. The best of these combine geranium, lavender and sandalwood, which all have a regulating effect on sebum secretion.

I have found the best results come from combining regular scalp massage with applications or rinses. Massaging the scalp each morning with two tablespoons of warmed pure unroasted sesame oil has an effect very quickly. Work the warmed oil into the scalp as you would a shampoo, using the heels of your hands to make small circular movements covering the whole of the scalp. If you don't mind slicked hair you can leave the oil on; otherwise shampoo off with a mild, frequent-use or herbal shampoo.

Every third day, make a horsetail rinse by pouring at least 1.2 litre (2 pints) of boiling water over 50–75g (2–3oz) of horsetail. Leave to steep for about a minute, then remove the herbs from the liquid. Once it has cooled sufficiently, rinse the hair thoroughly with it. Used over a period of about six weeks, this should prove a complete answer to dandruff and it can be repeated should the condition recur. I would advise paying attention to your diet and redressing any longstanding vitamin or mineral deficiency. One of the easiest ways to do this is to take a full-spectrum, yeast-free vitamin and mineral supplement and eat five portions of fresh fruit and vegetables every day. You may also consider consulting a naturopath or natural healthcare practitioner for a detailed health assessment and to confirm your nutritional status. They will also be able to recommend a supplement to suit your needs.

Dandruff may also be part of the body's response to a yeast infection (see **Athlete's Foot**), and diet is one of the major treatment choices if this is the case. Cutting down on sugar in all its forms and all foods containing yeast will have a positive effect on general health even if you don't have a yeast infection, and may improve the dandruff too.

Yeast-containing Foods

ALL breads including pitta bread (but not matzos, chappatis and some soda and rye breads). All foods containing or coated in breadcrumbs.

Yeast-enriched cakes, buns and pizza bases. All dairy products except milk, fresh rindless cheeses and un-salted butter. Yeast extract spreads such as Marmite, Bovril and Vegemite, vegetable pâtés and most stock cubes. Malt and malted drinks, vinegar and all pickled foods, soy sauce and all fermented foods and drinks such as wine and beer. Any fruit with a 'bloom', and all commercially prepared fruit juices, and those made including the skin of the fruit. Mushrooms and other mycoproteins. All foods containing the preservative monosodium glutamate (MSG). Vitamin products may contain yeast, or yeast-derived vitamin B and selenium. Double check the labels on all prepared foods.

Sugar-containing Foods

ALL types of sugar (white, demerara, muscovado, cane, etc.), golden syrup, molasses, treacle, and all cakes, sweet biscuits, puddings etc. containing sugar. Honey, jam, maple syrup, malt, ice cream, soft drinks, fruit juices and squashes and dried fruit. Most breads, chocolate, and a host of other prepared foods – check the labels. Medicines, which contain sugar in the form of syrups.

DEPRESSION

Clinical depression always requires an individual diagnosis and individual treatment. There are, however, some wonderful natural treatments that can help with the symptoms of both diagnosed illness and 'the blues'. In my experience, people suffering with depression do respond to a variety of treatments, including regular reflexology sessions, healing, aromatherapy, massage, Shamanism, and shiatsu. This all goes to prove that each individual will respond in different ways, and it is well worth exploring a range of supportive therapies until you find the most effective one for you.

Aromatherapy can help lighten your mood, and the regular use of essential oils in the bath, as a room scent and for massage can have a profound effect on the emotions. Jasmine is the oil of choice for depression, and its uplifting, softening, joy-bringing effects can be felt immediately. This is one of the more expensive essential oils, yet a drop or two will go a long way. The effect can be enhanced by growing the beautiful flowering plant close to a window, or even in a pot indoors. Other oils can also help – sandalwood and ylang ylang have a slight sedative effect as well as being anti-depressants. Sandalwood will also help you find the courage you need, through its effect on the kidney region, and ylang ylang can help with self-esteem and confidence. Geranium and rose both help lift a mood without any sedative effect and can be useful if fatigue is a problem and there is a feeling of down-heartedness.

The Bach flower remedies (if tolerated), can also help. Taking a few drops on waking, before going to bed, and at least twice more during the day is a useful pattern to follow and delivers an effective therapeutic lift. There are remedies for loneliness, lack of interest, and uncertainty, plus a range aimed specifically at despondency or despair. From these I find Oak a tremendous giver of strength and stability. Pine is most suitable for the peacemakers among us who will take enormous loads on to their own shoulders and often carry the blame for others, while Crab Apple, which is the remedy of cleansing, can help with the elimination of negative thoughts and energies. One of the easiest ways to take a mix of remedies is to add a few drops of each one to a small bottle of still mineral water. This can be kept in the fridge, and you can easily take it with you if you go out. It makes it a lot easier than measuring from a selection of remedy bottles each time a dose is taken. Some people may prefer to take Bach flower remedies externally because of their alcohol content (see pages 7–8).

Nutrition can play an important role in keeping endocrine and blood sugar levels at an optimum balance. In particular, supplementation with the B vitamins and zinc can show good results. It is important to rule out food intolerance or allergy as a cause or aggravator of the depression. One of the best ways to do this is to keep a diet diary (see page 23) for six weeks and see whether there are any connections between food and mood. It is also important not to rely on stimulants such as caffeine. Although these may appear to give a short-term lift to both humour and energy levels, they may mask symptoms and even interfere with your health in the long term.

The positive effects of sunshine need not be forgotten – some depressions are related to lack of sun. Apart from the biological effects of sunlight, simply being out and about in the natural world is uplifting, and the regular habit of going out for a walk, preferably in nature, or even just sitting on a park bench so long as it is in the sunshine, will have a cheering effect. You might also like to consider moonbathing – going out for a walk, or just to sit, in moonlight can stir powerful feelings.

Dramatic benefits in treating depression can be gained from developing an awareness of our own individual behavioural needs and activities. To this end, many forms of dynamic psychotherapy or active spirituality can transform the negativity of what can be perceived as a mundane existence. What many psychologists call motivation and purpose can also be termed hope, and in depression anything that can offer hope and encourage the person to take an interest in the outcome of things will have a positive effect. Somebody once said that you make plans on the good days, then on the bad days all you need to do is follow them. It is well worth finding a sympathetic practitioner with whom to make plans and follow them through.

DERMATITIS

This means any inflammation or irritation of the skin and is often used to describe a skin problem where the cause is unknown. Sensitivity to substances that come into contact with the skin is often an immediate cause, although overall health and stress levels can also be factors.

Each day we come into contact with an incredible number of substances, both natural and synthetic. I have a mild contact allergy to new rubber gloves: every time I put on a new pair I develop a tiny, painless rash all over my hands that disappears after the first day. I have been told by shop assistants, store managers and even some manufacturers that there is nothing in the rubber that could cause such an effect, and it took many months before I finally got somebody to admit that it could be narrowed down to one of two chemicals. One is added to the rubber during processing and the other and most likely culprit is the dusting which is put inside every new pair. The moral here is that although psychological factors will always play a part in our personal response to things, our individual physiology makes a difference too. (And there is something to be said for persistence – if you react to something and you're told there is nothing that could possibly be causing it, keep on until you find out the truth!)

A number of natural substances can also provoke skin reactions in some people, poison ivy and nettle rash are two obvious examples. A common allergic reaction to eating shellfish is a small but widespread red rash. (Here though it must be said that these animals are scavengers who tend to eat things on the ocean floor. This is where we dump poisons, nuclear byproducts, chemicals and sewage, so it could perhaps be another type of allergy.)

Soaps, detergents, new clothes, chemical cleaners, periods

spent in the garden, and diet are among the things it is worth scrutinising. Also remember that the dermatitis could be a response to seasonal changes such as the first pollen of the season or other airborne irritants, so think about the week before the irritation appeared and relive it in minute detail if necessary, to see if any cause can be found.

Whatever the cause, sore, red or dry skin will often respond to a treatment plan of oatmeal baths (see **Eczema**), nettle tea and calendula cream. Drinking up to three cups of nettle tea per day will help cleanse you from the inside out, and treating any particularly sore spots with a thin covering of calendula cream should clear any difficulties within two days. If they persist, help should be sought from a naturopath or natural healthcare practitioner.

DIARRHOEA

The best cure for diarrhoea is to eat dry matzos. Take two if possible, with a cup of warm water, although you may feel that one of these large wheat crackers is enough, and repeat after three hours. Once the gut has emptied completely, a cup of liquorice tea or of Vata blend – a special herbal mix available from Ayurvedic suppliers (see page 147) – taken every two hours will settle the system. Do not eat anything else during that day – give your body time to adjust after the shock of the upset – but make sure you drink plenty of warm water. If you find your energy levels are very low, adding a small teaspoon of raw honey to each cup of warm water should do the trick.

Be especially gentle with yourself over the next day or so, and particularly with your gut. Regular cups of Vata blend or liquorice tea, and warm, gentle, nursery food like soups and puréed or mashed vegetables, eaten regularly, will help sustain energy levels and soothe the nerves. Some fennel seeds eaten after each meal will help with digestion. A few drops of Dr Bach's Rescue Remedy, if tolerated, can be taken up to five times a day once the diarrhoea has stopped. The drops can be rubbed on to the pulse spots on your wrists and neck, if preferred.

Diarrhoea is usually a sign that your body needed to expel immediately something that it did not want. It is an emergency action, and not something that should occur on a regular basis. If it does, you would do well to consult a naturopath or natural healthcare practitioner.

DIZZINESS

Dizziness can have any number of causes, from standing up too quickly to an inner ear infection, and it is a good reason for consulting your naturopath or natural healthcare practitioner if it occurs regularly. It is quite a common reaction to any form of cleansing or detoxification regime and if you are following one of these it is a good idea to take this as a sign that you need to increase the speed of elimination. Your practitioner will be able to help you with this, and one of the most effective ways is to double the amount of good clean water that you drink and take up to 2g of vitamin C with bioflavonoids each day.

Dropping your head forward very slightly, so that your chin is just moving towards your chest, and stretching up as high as you can with both arms, is the best instant cure I know. Hold this position for two minutes and repeat if necessary, although it rarely is.

Great care must be taken with the next remedy, but it has a wonderful effect on recurrent dizziness. Take 20 green mistletoe leaves and liquidise them or put them through a juice extractor. Take one tablespoon twice a day. The care must be taken when picking the leaves to ensure that no berries, which are poisonous, are picked along with them. Autumn is the best season for gathering mistletoe leaves.

EARACHE

Warmth is always of great help in soothing and healing earache. Lying on one side with your head on a hot-water bottle is one of the best ways to get off to sleep and can be very soothing at any time of day. Another, older method of holding heat around the ear and the jaw is to make a small flannel bag (the size of a large teabag) and fill it about three-quarters full with rock salt. Place this in a hot oven until heated right through, and then lay it on a thin cotton handkerchief and place on the ear. Hold it there until cooled, and then repeat.

Nowadays, Hopi ear candles are widely available. These are by far the best treatment for a full range of ear troubles and they also help with headaches, sinus complaints, adenoid and inner ear problems. This traditional North American Indian method draws infection and negative energies out of the body more effectively than any other. Hopi ear candles can be obtained from a number of traders in traditional American wares and some health-food shops (see page 147 for suppliers). They are best used following the instructions that come with them.

A few drops of a strong, warmed infusion of fresh marjoram can be dropped into the outer ear several times a day to help dissolve any build-up of wax. To make the marjoram infusion, cram a small mug or teacup full of fresh leaves and cover with boiling water. Leave to stand until tepid, then strain, reserving the liquid. You may also soak a pad of cotton in the liquid and use it as a compress (see page 5) for the outer ear and jaw area. The leaves may be placed in a muslin bag and added to the bathwater for a relaxing and sedating aid to insomnia – an important consideration if pain from the ear is troublesome.

For localised irritation of the ears, a small amount of warmed almond oil, a wonderfully soothing substance, may be dropped into the outer ear. Great care must always be taken when putting anything into the ear, and particular attention paid to check the temperature of the oil before it is applied.

ECZEMA

This red rash can appear anywhere on the body. It is most often accompanied by scaling and blisters and is extremely itchy. If scratched, it often starts to weep, and areas may then become infected. The itchiness is one of the worst aspects of this skin condition and may cause sleepless nights.

Although commonly regarded as an illness in its own right, eczema rarely occurs without other symptoms and is often the result of supressed childhood illnesses. The skin reflects the condition of the lungs and the liver, and eczema often appears when the body is having difficulty coping with stress, and before or after breathing difficulties such as asthma and hayfever.

A very successful long-term treatment for eczema sufferers is to follow a detoxification programme and take specific supplements to tone the liver. Beetroot is an excellent liver tonic and should be eaten raw every day. Dandelion coffee has a similar astringent effect and may be drunk daily as a substitute for ordinary coffee. Eliminating all cow's products from the diet, and avoiding wheat, yeast and sugar (see page 74) will make it easier for the body's digestive system and show in improved skin condition. Strong seasonings such as chilli, mustard and black pepper need to be avoided, too.

One cup of an infusion of burdock root should be taken each day, while exercise and time spent in the fresh air should be increased to speed healing. Two cups of nettle tea per day will help with overall elimination as well as soothing the skin.

If the eczema affects only very small areas, the following recipe should help. It can be applied twice daily and has tremendous healing ability. Mix together seven drops each of soluble vitamin A, E, and evening primrose oil and add sufficient vitamin C powder and pure unroasted sesame oil to mix into a paste. Spread the paste thinly on the sore spots and leave open to the air. This is also an excellent skin food for delicate areas such as the face that have been exposed to too much sun or wind.

Light pure unroasted sesame oil may be used as a massage oil (see page 4) to cover the affected areas and can be applied as often as required, although once a day is usually sufficient. A few drops of essential oil of rose may be added to the sesame oil and has a very strong healing effect.

Oatmeal Bath

For overall relief, however widespread the problem, take a hot oat bath. Place 500g (1lb) mixed oatflakes and oatmeal in a muslin bag or a thin cotton handkerchief and tie it to the hot tap while running the bath. Make the tie long enough for the bag to soak in the bath once it has filled. This is very soft and soothing for the skin and has strong curative properties. These baths can be taken as often as desired, and you will probably see an improvement after just one.

If discomfort is severe, apply a little grated fresh horseradish root that has been steeped in some natural yoghurt in the fridge for an hour. This will cool and soothe straight away and only has beneficial effects in terms of local healing, so may be repeated as often as you like.

CHI DYNAMICS CLEANSING EXERCISE

There is a lovely Chi dynamics exercise which is both cleansing and invigorating. It can be done in combination with the other Chi dynamics exercises in this book (see pages 43 and 71) or on its own, and may be repeated as often as feels good.

Stand with your knees soft, or slightly bent, arms by your sides, and imagine a small pool of cool, calm water just beside your left foot. Without moving your feet, rotate your body so that you are facing the pool and drop down towards it by bending your knees. Reach forward to scoop up some of this water with your hands. Don't worry if you can't reach down to the floor; this is a magic pool and you can reach it from any level so long as you are doing your best.

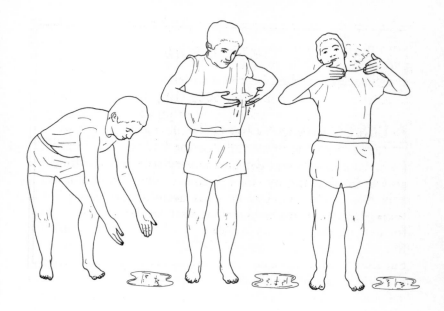

Gather up an armful of the healing water and bring it up the left side of your body, straightening up as you do so. Draw the water up the outside of the thigh, up over the hip and the left breast to the face. You will find your weight drops onto your right leg. Then lean back slightly, splashing your face with the soothing water. Once you have practised this it will be easy to do with one large inhalation. Then let your breath out with a whoosh as the water runs from your face. Sweep the water from your body with your hands as it falls back down to the earth, carrying any negativity and impurity with it. Let your weight roll back onto your left leg as you push the water away.

Pause for just a moment and feel yourself to be a little lighter, a little easier and refreshed, and then return to the start position. Repeat the exercise three more times.

Turn to your right and do the same thing for the right side of your body, gently bending down to raise the water up the right thigh, over the right hip and up over the right breast to your face, from where it may cascade down the body, cleansing as it goes. Repeat this three more times, working with your breath if you can – breathing in as you gather the water and carry it up and over your body, and then out as it falls and cleanses your body – and then relax.

EYESTRAIN AND SORE EYES

Eyebright cream can safely be applied around the whole eye area and brings speedy relief. This soothing, clear gel is available from herbalist suppliers and health-food shops. Cold used peppermint tea bags and cucumber slices are both good for placing on closed eyes while you lie down and relax for five to 15 minutes. Ordinary tea bags are useful for this too, but they tend to have an astringent effect on the skin around the eyes so are best used over a smear of protective cream or gel, such as Vaseline, calendula ointment or unroasted sesame oil.

Much soreness and strain can be eased by regularly varying the focus of your eyes. This simply means looking up from whatever you are doing at least every 15 minutes and looking around the room, out of the window, down at your fingernails and then back to your work. These simple manoeuvres will relax the eyes, and it is a good idea to do them while relaxing, reading or watching television as well as at work. A useful exercise to strengthen the focus is to hold a sharpened pencil in front of your face with the point held up at eye level. Slowly bring the pencil in until it is touching the end of your nose, keeping the point of the pencil in focus all the time, and then move it back out to its original place. Repeat this exercise several times each day.

Often tired eyes simply need a rest, and covering them with your hands for five minutes at a time (see **Conjuctivitis**) will supply the darkness and the warmth necessary to revitalise and clear them.

A chamomile compress applied at the end of the day will soothe and heal tired eyes and help heal any bloodshot or dryness. Add a large teaspoon of chamomile flowers to 300ml (½ pint) of boiling milk. Leave it for about a minute and then strain. When the liquid is hand hot, soak a cotton handker-chief or thin cotton tea-towel in it, wring it dry and place over the eyes. Leave in place until cool.

FAINTING

There is no natural reason why anyone should faint, so if this happens frequently or with no apparent cause a full health check is advised. Someone who has fainted as a response to a sudden physical or emotional shock will soon come round if they can be placed in a position that encourages blood flow to the head. As people usually fall down when they faint, this is quite easily done. If you feel you are about to faint, sitting down with your head between your knees for five minutes may well be enough to prevent it. Otherwise, lying down flat with your eyes covered to shut out all the light works well.

Essential oil of lemon grass has a wonderfully grounding scent. You can place it under the nose of someone recovering from a faint and also add it to an oil burner after the episode to allow the aroma to keep on working for a while.

A cup of hot peppermint tea with a little honey added will help get the person stabilised again, and of course Dr Bach's Rescue Remedy (if tolerated) can be taken every half hour and rubbed on the pulse spots in the wrists and temples.

Another effective way to settle the system and hasten recovery is to take a tablespoon of Swedish bitters (if toler-ated) dissolved in a glass of water. It is said that if a few drops are applied neat to the lips of a person who is in a faint they will come round straight away. I have never tried this but can attest to the wonderful effects of this mixture in all manner of situations.

Comfort, reassurance and the caring touch of another per-son will help to settle someone who has just fainted, and even using a gentle tone of voice will have a positive effect.

If you are recovering from a faint, take things slowly and very carefully for the rest of the day, having a nap or at least getting a very early night. Make sure you stay warm and have plenty of warm drinks.

Stone Breathing

HOLDING a stone to the energy centre just below your navel while taking slow, deep breaths will settle you within minutes after a faint. There is no need to have a special stone, just find one from anywhere around you and let the stone's relationship with the earth remind you of your need to feel more grounded. Take the stone in your left hand and place it on your abdomen, just below your navel. Cover it with your right hand and try to feel the strength and solidity of the stone sharing itself with you as you breathe long, slow, steady breaths. Keep it in place until you feel quite solid and then return it to the place where you found it.

FATIGUE

Fatigue can have any number of causes, ranging from a natural response to over-exertion to a symptom of allergies or a reaction to stress or illness. If it is a long-standing complaint, or occurs after a virus such as flu, it is a good idea to consult a naturopath or other natural healthcare practitioner for a full health check.

The regular addition of some form of sea vegetable or seaweed to the diet will help keep the thyroid in good working order. Kelp may be taken as a supplement in capsule or tablet form, or even better, choose from some of the wide range of sea vegetables, such as sea cucumber and seaweeds like dulse, arame, wakame, nori and carageen and eat them each day with meals. Sea vegetables can be found in dried form in health-food shops and many oriental groceries, and those lucky enough to live near clean areas of coastline may taste them. A daily supplement of 50mg of co-enzyme Q helps generate

Fenugreek Pick-me-up

For a fast-acting pick-me-up, put one tablespoon of fenugreek seeds and three cups of water in a non-aluminium pan that isn't non-stick and simmer for five minutes. Add blackstrap molasses to taste (ideally no less than a teaspoon and no more than a tablespoon) and drink one cup a day. This age-old Middle Eastern tonic is particularly effective for women, who benefit most from its iron and mineral content. It can be a delicious drink, so it is worth experimenting with the amount of fenugreek seeds and the simmering time – generally the longer it is simmered the milder the fenugreek flavour.

energy at a cellular level. Although the results may take a while to show they can often be surprising.

Wheatgrass juice is another valuable tonic, made by juicing grown or sprouted wheatberries. A glass of this taken each day has marked revitalising qualities. If it is not available but you have a juicer, adding fresh green leaves such as lettuce to your juice will have a similar, though less potent, effect.

Relief from mental fatigue can be gained by adding a few drops of essential oil of rosemary to an oil burner and keeping it on a desk or table near you. Rosemary helps sharpen the mental faculties and heighten memory, so it is a perfect study aid.

Often the best remedies for fatigue are sleep and variety. A short nap will often take the edge off things enough to enable you to cope until bedtime. Fatigue may be a sign that the body is either tired or bored, and giving it a short rest or a little variety will acknowledge that you are listening to it but cannot respond fully just yet. It is a source of great pleasure to me how the body will become revitalised and seem completely changed if you switch to a different activity. This is especially true if movement is involved. Going for a short walk, and getting out amongst nature is always revitalising, but moving to another chair, taking a walk once round the office or home, or turning up the radio and dancing for a few minutes, will all work. It is as if we get stuck in a rut and even the simplest change will re-energise us and replace any lost enthusiasm. As a final word, the body *needs* time to rest and repair itself, and if you are recovering from illness or sickness it will require more sleep than usual.

FEVER

Raising its temperature is often the body's way of fighting disease. It knows that viruses and bacteria will often be killed off at a lower temperature than you will, so having a fever seems like a very sensible thing to do. Problems only occur if the person is very young or old, or physically depleted. If this is the case, professional advice should be sought straight away.

In a normally healthy person if the temperature does not rise above 101 degrees for more than a day there should be no problems. Make sure they are in a well-ventilated but draught-free room and have lots to drink. Don't worry if the appetite dissappears; it is best not to make the body work at digesting food at this time because it will be concentrating all its energy on fighting a battle on the immune front. One of the effects of a high temperature is that you will be obliged to rest in bed, and without the demands of everyday life the body can get on with the job in hand much more readily. Knowing this, it is really senseless to try and 'struggle on' or work through a high temperature – follow your body's lead and go to bed.

Quinine is very good at reducing fever, so if you need to cool down or the temperature has been raised for a long time, a small glass of tonic water taken every two hours will often be enough to reduce it. Chamomile tea can have a similar effect; try sipping a cup of the hot tea twice each day.

Foot Wrap

If a fever is suspected – often symptoms can be detected the night before, particularly if you have a cold coming on – the following hydrotherapy measure will help. Get a pair of long cotton socks and soak them in cold water containing two capfuls of apple cider vinegar. Wring them out and put them on before going to bed, leaving them on through the night. Your legs and feet can be further wrapped with small towels to protect the bedclothes, or a large plastic bin bag can be used to cover the sheets.

Apart from its therapeutic effects, this is so comforting once it is in place that a good night's sleep is almost assured. The socks will need to be removed when you wake up, and your legs and feet washed. (If you don't have enough energy to take a shower or bath, gentle rinsing in a footbath or plastic bowl will be fine).

Try to take things easy for a few days after a fever. Make sure to get extra rest and fresh air, and try to take a little gentle exercise out in nature, such as a short walk in the park. Follow the cleansing diet on page 20 and don't worry if you don't feel like eating very much at all for the first few days. After this, if your appetite has not returned, add a small slice of fresh ginger root the size of your little fingertip to a cup of hot water and sip it half an hour before mealtimes. This will be gently warming for the digestion and encourage your appetite. You may also like to try the Body Pack on page 14. This will provide an overall boost to your constitution as well as reduce the fever and help you to feel better.

FLATULENCE

Air in the body has a natural tendency to rise, so sitting up straight when you're eating or, if it is too late for that, getting down on to all fours and dropping your chest down so that your bottom is sticking up in the air, will help relieve some of the discomfort of accumulated gas.

Taking two tablets of naturally activated charcoal with meals will resolve the problem immediately but the charcoal will absorb just about everything else, including the nutrients in the food, so this cannot be taken more than once a week. Drinking a small glass of very fizzy water such as Perrier a few minutes after eating should shift any upper digestive air-locks.

Follow the advice for **Indigestion** and eat in a calm, unhurried manner. Also, try to ensure that you chew your food thoroughly and take care when eating and talking that you give eating precedence. When we hurry it is very easy to swallow air along with the food, and then if the food isn't well masticated digestive difficulties may swiftly follow.

If nothing else works, this nasty-tasting remedy is truly effective. Crush a peeled garlic clove directly into a cup of hot water and sip it after each meal in place of tea or coffee.

GINGIVITIS

This is an inflammation of the gums surrounding the teeth. There is no evidence of this problem at all in people who eat an exclusively wholefood diet without sugar; indeed Stone Age people appeared to have better mouth health and fewer holes in their teeth than people today. Sugar is the main culprit, allowing the build-up in the mouth of a sticky substance called dextran which adheres to the base of the teeth and allows plaque to form. Refined foods can leave residues in the mouth which then provide the perfect fuel for the plaque to ferment. Nutritional status also plays a big part; if you follow a wholefood diet and eat five portions of fresh fruit and vegetables each day, the high nutrient levels you build up will go a long way towards preventing gum disease.

The mouth is regularly flushed clean when we swallow and when we eat and drink. It responds relatively quickly to changes in environment, and although the advice above is mainly preventative, you will find your oral health improves if you embark upon it straight away.

Rubbing the gums gently with some fresh parsley leaves is a good way of introducing vitamin C straight to the site where it is needed and also has a soothing effect on the inflamed tissue. Flat-leaved parsley is easier to use, although a small bunch of curly parsley with do just as well.

Rinsing the mouth each night with a cooled infusion of lemon verbena helps prevent overnight decay in the teeth and is also good for the gums. Cover a bunch of fresh lemon verbena leaves with boiling water, leave to stand until cool and then strain. The leaves can be returned to the garden for compost or used as part of a soothing balm for blisters and shingles. The liquor will keep in a fridge for three days.

During the day the mouth may be rinsed with a solution of warm water to which has been added two drops of tincture of myrrh. This antiseptic wash can be used before and after each meal and at other times to give some relief from tenderness or pain.

GOUT

See **Arthritis**.

HAEMORRHOIDS

Haemorrhoids, or piles, are really varicose veins in the bottom. They can cause a lot of pain with each bowel movement and may bleed and protrude from the anus. Applying a hot compress (see page 5) before the bowel movement, if possible, and having an iced water spray to hand for use immediately afterwards will help with pain relief and in the long term should reduce both bleeding and protrusion.

Sitz Bath

THE best cure for haemorrhoids is to have a daily sitz bath. You will need a bath and a large container such as a tub, galvanised bath or baby bath to place inside it. Fill the bath with hot water and the container with cold. Sit with your bottom in the hot bath, bend your knees, and place your feet in the cold water of the container for two minutes, then change over so that your feet are in the hot bath and you are sitting in the container of cold water. Stay there for about another two minutes and then change around again. Repeat this three times, ending with your bottom in the cold water. Ideally the water should completely cover your pelvis and the top of your thighs, and it will help if you slosh the water around to ensure it moves between your legs.

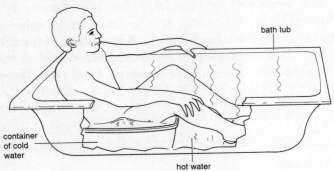

bath tub

container of cold water

hot water

Dry yourself briskly with a towel and rest quietly for a few minutes. This is a dramatically effective technique for relieving all sorts of pelvic difficulties and it may leave you feeling a little tired afterwards. A short rest should be sufficient to allow you to feel the powerfully energising effects of the bath.

Keep the stool as soft as possible by increasing your intake of raw vegetables, fruit and neutral fluids, such as water, herbal teas and fruit and vegetable juices. People often increase the amount of bran in their diet but this needs to be accompanied by a dramatic increase in the amount of water drunk (at least an extra 2 pints each day) to have a positive effect.

Vitamin C is very effective for wound healing and a supplement of 500mg three times a day with meals could be taken to good effect. Smoking is a particular irritant for the bowel, as well as destroying vitamin C, so it is well to avoid or at least cut down on cigarettes during acute episodes.

Slant board exercises (see page 18) are of great benefit when dealing with haemorrhoids and may be practised up to three times a day. This is a very easy thing to set up in the home and the benefits are enormous. Another useful measure is to raise the foot of the bed by about 10cm (4 inches) by placing a few telephone directories or similar sturdy books underneath the legs.

If the pain is great, apply powdered goldenseal mixed with fresh aloe vera gel to the affected area for immediate relief. Alternatively, moisten a wad of cotton wool with Swedish bitters and place it at the entrance to the anus. Secure in place with a plaster and leave on overnight. The astringent effect should carry through to the first bowel movement of the day.

HAIR LOSS

See **Alopecia**.

HALITOSIS

Halitosis, or bad breath, can be caused by a number of factors, usually originating either in the mouth or in the digestive system. Good oral hygiene is an important preventative measure, and will help reduce the incidence of gum disease and dental decay, both potential causes of bad breath.

Brush your teeth thoroughly at night, because unpleasant morning breath can often be traced to the breakdown of bacteria that has been in the mouth all night. The continual production and swallowing of saliva act as a mini mouthwash, but throughout the night any food matter left lodged between the teeth or around the gums will remain there. You might also consider whether your toothpaste has sugar in it – as many of them do – which means that you are coating your teeth with sugar solution before going to sleep. I have never understood how dentists and oral hygienists can recommend this.

Bad breath may be a sign of a sluggish digestion, putrefaction of foods already in the gut or may be a symptom of constipation (see **Indigestion** and **Constipation**). If it is a constant problem, a complete cleansing programme is the best course of action. A three-day cleansing diet (see page 20) combined with some active skincare measures such as regular skin brushing (see page 17) and a weekly salt glow (see below) will help awaken the skin and bowel to the need for improved elimination.

Salt Glow

Put 1kg (2lb) of coarse sea salt in a bowl and add enough hot water to make a thick slush. Taking small handfuls, rub the mixture well into your whole body for a few minutes. Do not be too rough – the slush can be quite abrasive, particularly on more sensitive areas – but do be as vigorous as possible. Shower off with hot water and then follow that with water as cold as you can bear for another minute or so. This should leave your skin glowing and warm and will take a lot of pressures off the body's other eliminative routes.

A one-day juice or fresh fruit fast will have a regulating effect on the digestion and help relieve any internal build-ups that might be contributing to or causing the bad odour. If you undertake such a plan, make sure to drink lots of good, clean water and get a little extra rest. The best and most eliminative fruits for such a plan are pineapple, grapes and melon. In the meantime, chewing fresh parsley is a wonderful breath freshener and also means that you take in a little extra iron and vitamin C – no bad thing.

HANGOVERS

There seems to be a multitude of potential hangover cures, ranging from 'hair of the dog' to taking cold showers. Every individual will find what works best for them but there is a theory that protein, calcium and vitamin C make the most helpful combination.

After drinking alcohol, drink large amounts of water before going to bed. In the morning, take a buffered soluble vitamin C tablet on waking and follow it with a good breakfast, preferably one containing protein, calcium and vitamin C. If this sounds too much like a large meal, don't worry – the process of eating anything will have a positive effect on your system. Fresh beetroot juice is a wonderful liver tonic and by far the best thing to drink. You can make this yourself quite easily if you have a juice extractor, and it can be bought from health food shops. If you do have a juicer, try adding a few lettuce or dandelion leaves for extra chlorophyll.

If you can manage to make this 'morning cocktail', it certainly seems to clear the head. Mix together one cup each of pineapple and grapefruit juice, whip in half a cup of live goat's or sheep's milk yoghurt, add 1g vitamin C powder and then top up with half a cup of a strong sparkling mineral water such as Perrier.

A large mug of lemon water is a great way to begin every day, whatever happened the night before, because of its positive alkalinising effect on the system. Place a generous squeeze of lemon juice and a couple of slices of lemon in a mug, cover with cold water (this prevents the vitamin C from oxidising) and then top up with boiling water. Make sure that the lemon is organically grown, or at least that it has not been waxed.

HAYFEVER

This seasonal allergy can begin as early as the end of March with the first tree pollens and extend right through the summer. Constitutional work (see **Allergies**) does pay off, and pre-season preparation makes all the difference.

Burning the essential oils of chamomile and/or melissa will have a soothing effect and serve the dual purpose of moistening the air. Add a few drops of either of these oils to some pure unroasted sesame oil for massaging the back of the neck and shoulders too.

A sprig of rosemary or lavender, or a few drops of lavender or eucalyptus essential oils added to a handkerchief, will help keep the nasal passages clear. Stronger oils such as Olbas can be kept in reserve for later in the season when your tolerance of some of the herbs has increased.

A good cure for head congestion is to apply a raw onion poultice to the back of the neck before going to bed. Smear the skin with a dab of pure unroasted sesame oil or calendula cream and then add a strip of gauze or thin cotton, place some grated onion on top and wrap around in another piece of cotton fabric or a clean tea-towel. If you tie this around your neck like a scarf it should remain in place.

Extra sleep is important when you are suffering with hayfever because constantly reacting in this way is so physically wearying. Try to get an extra hour before midnight each night.

My mother's best piece of advice is to smear the rim of each nostril with a little Vaseline. It works wonders, seeming to 'catch' the pollen before it troubles the delicate nasal membranes. It does need repeating quite often, and certainly after blowing your nose. She also suggests hanging damp nets at the windows – this means they can be opened quite safely, a luxury on a day with a high pollen count.

The tissue salt Nat. Mur. is the most effective single remedy I know, although there is also a combination remedy on the market which many people speak highly of. Diet and supplements are equally important, and avoiding mucus-forming foods during the summer can have wonderful effects: try eliminating wheat and cow's products from your diet for three weeks. You could also take a daily dose of 0.2ml of echinacea tincture (if tolerated) and 2g of vitamin C to stimulate the immune system and help prevent further mucus irritation.

Humming

HUMMING is a very useful exercise if you have hayfever, clearing the nasal passages and also stimulating the sinuses as the resonance of each note moves through the head. Simply spending a few minutes humming each morning can tip the balance and leave you feeling better during the day. The humming sound also seems to have a soothing effect on the body's overall balance, and the deep breaths you need to take help improve your breathing generally. This is particularly important because many hayfever sufferers don't seem to take deep breaths at all between spring and autumn! Also practise relaxed diaphragmatic breathing (see page 25).

HEADACHES

There can be so many causes for headaches that it is a source of great wonder to me that nature has remedies for all of them. Headaches brought on by overtiredness due to lack of sleep will soon respond to a cup of rosehip tea sweetened with a spoonful of honey. Those caused through nervous tension or spending too long in a stuffy environment will pass if you sip a cup of very hot yarrow tea as slowly as possible.

A few drops of essential oil of lavender added to a tablespoon of pure unroasted sesame oil and massaged gently into the forehead and temples will help relieve the discomfort of sinus congestion and that 'muggy-headed' feeling. Simply crushing a few peppermint leaves on to the forehead will also have a stimulating and clearing effect. Placing a handkerchief soaked in any type of cool vinegar on the forehead will help clear congestion and sinus pain.

We often do not realise how little fresh air we have to breathe, and taking a walk in a wood or park, or even along a tree-lined avenue can soon clear a light headache. If going outdoors is not possible or the air quality is bad, one good exercise is to stand up and quite quickly make big circling movements with the arms. Bring both arms up more or less along the centre of the body and then let them swing out and round till they are by your sides, keeping the movement going for a few minutes. This opens up the chest and is really exhilarating.

Headaches that are caused by a gut disturbance or upset stomach will often disappear if you take one teaspoon of Swedish bitters (if tolerated) dissolved in half a cup of warm water before and after meals for one day. The headache that comes from a sluggish digestion can be eliminated by drinking a large glass of pineapple and grapefruit juice – the fresher the juices, the better.

One of the commonest causes of headaches is bowel congestion and any of the remedies for **Constipation** should help with this. If it is a regular problem, though, it is well worth undertaking some regular cleansing and detoxification of the system. Follow the three-day cleansing diet on page 20 and consider consulting a naturopath or natural healthcare practitioner.

Finally, chewing a small amount of the root of meadowsweet, an abundant plant, will give fast relief for most headaches.

HERPES

We tend to experience the herpes virus in one of three ways: as cold sores, genital herpes or herpes zoster, the relative of chickenpox that is also known as shingles. All three are more likely to occur when you are feeling run down or under stress. The effects of the virus in the system can be devastating, and alongside the pain and irritation from the sores or blisters it is not uncommon to experience lethargy, depression and a number of other wide-ranging symptoms. Supplements of B complex and 200iu of vitamin E each day will help the nervous system generally.

Cold sores on or around the mouth will soon disappear if a few drops of juice from an organically grown lemon are squeezed on to them several times a day. Tea-tree (or ti-tree) oil can also be used, applied neat on a piece of cotton wool or a cotton bud. (Do not take any essential oil internally.) I prefer using the lemon juice because it smells and tastes better, and there is the added benefit of the vitamin C.

Genital herpes can result in a number of problems, not least because the site of the lesions or blisters may not be easily treatable. Women who have been exposed to genital herpes are recommended to have cervical smear tests at least once a year. If the blisters can be seen, regular applications of neat tea-tree essential oil will sting, but can help relieve the itching and aches that often accompany the eruption.

A cold compress of goat's milk yoghurt can be applied for up to 30 minutes at a time, six times a day. The easiest way to do this is to cover a sanitary towel with the yoghurt and then just wear it as normal. After each application, rinse the whole area with cold water and gently pat dry. Then apply a mixture of equal parts of bergamot and eucalyptus essential oils – this is one of the rare occasions when they are applied directly – or equal parts of goldenseal, skullcap and lobelia tinctures. It is possible to alternate both these mixtures until you find which one suits you best.

Large amounts of vitamin C, echinacea tincture (if tolerated) and fresh garlic should be included in your diet, which should otherwise be as simple as possible. Follow the cleansing diet on page 20, or restrict your diet to rice and steamed or lightly cooked vegetables throughout an attack. If you can tolerate it, take 0.2ml of echinacea tincture twice a day and 1g of vitamin C with each meal.

An imbalance in the amino acids lysine and arginine may precipitate attacks, so take a lysine supplement of at least 500mg daily. At the same time, avoid foods rich in arginine. These include nuts, gelatine, chocolate, carob, coconut, seeds, oats, lentils and all pulses, brown rice, peas and onions. These dietary rules may need to be adhered to for several months but they have been shown to be very successful.

Shingles is best treated by following a juice-only diet consisting of fresh fruit and vegetable juices plus water and herbal teas until the worst of the pain and other symptoms have disappeared. If this takes longer than three days, however, consult your naturopath or natural healthcare practitioner. Combine this with cold water showers all over the affected area and repeated applications of Swedish bitters. Alternatively, make a mixture of equal parts of chamomile, sage and sweet clover, two parts of oats and half a part of lady's mantle. Cover with 1.2 litres (2 pints) of water and bring to the boil, then remove from the heat and leave to stand for five minutes. Strain, reserving the herbs, and use the liquid as a wash for the affected area. Wash several times daily or, if it is too painful, apply with a very soft paintbrush. The herbs can be placed on a light bandage and worn as a pack overnight.

With all these hydrotherapy measures it is important to ensure that fresh clean towels are always used and that these are not shared with anybody else.

HICCOUGHS

Every family seems to have its own cure for hiccoughs. I always get the best results by drinking half a cup of water from the wrong side of the cup. Swallowing 12 times in succession, an act that requires a lot of concentration, works well too.

Other solutions include holding your breath, swallowing some mustard, or having someone drop a cold key down your back. One of the easiest things to try is pressing the thumb of your right hand into the palm of the left and holding your breath at the same time. If that doesn't work, swallowing a teaspoon of vinegar (any type) should do the trick!

Finally by far the tastiest remedy of all, the following is especially useful if the hiccoughs have lasted for a long time, and is very popular with children of all ages. Mix together two tablespoons of fresh grated coconut and two tablespoons of thick set honey. Roll the mixture into small balls and chew one at a time. They are thick, concentrated and delicious, and I don't know why they work but they do.

Hives

See **Urticaria**.

Indigestion

The term indigestion covers a range of complaints from wind (see **Flatulence**) to pain and general discomfort. A key aspect of being able to digest meals is having the time and the right atmosphere in which to do so. Many indigestion sufferers will respond to relaxation, to taking time to eat in congenial surroundings with good friends or family, or alone away from bustle and noise. A gentle stroll or a lie-down for five minutes after a meal will all help the digestive process. Sitting up while you eat is also important – the 'couch potato' syndrome of eating while slouched in a chair and then not moving for hours is a recipe for digestive complaints.

The amount and type of food we eat also influences how well we manage to process our meals. There are occasions when we know we are eating too much or the wrong type of food (fat is hardest of all to digest), or even when we are emotionally upset and have a sense that eating is not the right thing to do. It pays to listen to the body at such times, and if this means skipping a meal or delaying it, travelling a little further to find a more suitable restaurant, or deciding to cook more oneself, then that is a lot easier than dealing with ill health.

Simple measures such as instigating a regular pattern for mealtimes will do a lot to settle the body's digestive function. Most people do best if they eat their largest meal in the middle of the day and have only a light supper.

Eating a few fennel seeds after each meal or adding them to the main course will improve digestion and help with any burping afterwards. Dill has a protective effect on the stomach and can be added freely to a number of meals. It is used as the basis for gripe water, which has a wonderfully settling effect on children. (The name dill comes from the Saxon name 'dilla', which means to lull, and it has a softening, quieting influence on digestion.) Charcoal tablets will do the same and can be a great help with flatulence, but as they absorb nutrients they are not to be recommended as a regular supplement. I find that a small glass of very fizzy water such as Perrier will do the same job if drunk immediately after the meal, not with it.

On the Continent it is common to take a *digestif* after eating, and in Spain chamomile tea is the most popular. This is a great settler and will soothe and calm the most troublesome of stomachs. Anise and other liqueurs tend to be effective because of the seeds they use rather than for their alcohol content.

Food combining is a system that works well for a number of people, at least for a period of time. This consists of separating meals into protein-based and carbohydrate-based ones and eating them with the right accompaniments. Try eating one correctly combined meal each day to see whether it has an effect on your symptoms, or try switching completely to this way of eating for six weeks and then assess the overall change. There are many books available giving detailed information and food-combining lists (see Further Reading, page 151).

It is well worth experimenting to find the style of eating that works best for you. Some people need a glass of warm water with their meal to ease digestion; others do best if they do not drink anything at all for up to half an hour after a meal. Seasonal influences will also make a difference, colouring not just our appetite but also the way we like to eat.

Naturopathy, Ayurvedic medicine and Chinese herbalism are among the many systems of healthcare that offer alternative ways of dealing with our nutritional needs. If you are eating the foods that suit you in a way that is right for you, indigestion should not really be a problem.

INFECTED CUTS, ETC.

Small gashes or skin punctures can be covered with a bread poultice, which will draw out any possible infection very quickly. Prepare the poultice by cutting the crusts off three slices of wholemeal bread and then covering the bread with boiling water. Mash the water and bread together into a paste, place this in a clean tea-towel or strip of cotton fabric, then squeeze out any surplus water and apply the poultice as hot as you can possibly bear. Leave it on for about ten minutes, and then replace it. This can be left in place for up to three hours, and then you can apply another fresh poultice.

INGROWN TOENAILS

It is important to cut the toenails as straight as possible so there is little risk of a cut corner or rounded edge being encouraged to grow into the side of the toe itself. After filing with an emery board (not a metal file) to remove any rough edges, make two strong abrasive movements in the corner of the nail on the nail surface. If you do this each time you cut your toenails, the ingrown part will grow out within about three months (see page 104).

If the ingrown toenails are causing pain, bathing the feet regularly in warm salty water can be very soothing. Add a handful of sea salt crystals to a footbath full of warm water and soak the feet till the water cools. This can be repeated daily. Dr Bach's Rescue Remedy cream may also be applied to the affected area after bathing, and this should considerably reduce any discomfort.

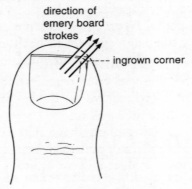

direction of
emery board
strokes

ingrown corner

INSECT BITES AND STINGS

Dock leaves are an old country remedy for nettle stings and it is said that wherever there are nettles growing, dock will not be far away. Other widely found remedies are lemon balm and plantain – the leaves from either will soothe the skin after insect bites. Take care to rinse them before use in case they have been exposed to pollutants and to minimise the risk of transferring bacteria.

At home, a slice of fresh onion will bring instant relief if placed on the site of a sting. Dilute vinegar of any type is useful for wasp stings and dilute bicarbonate of soda soothes after a bee has stung. (Remember vinegar for 'vasps', bicarb for bees.)

Burning dried sage is a useful way of deterring insects – they seem to dislike both the smoke and the sage itself – and a few drops of essential oil of lavender added to the water in an oil burner has much the same effect. This essential oil may also be added to a carrier oil and applied to the body to deter mosquitoes and other flying insects. An easy way to do this is to soak a small piece of cotton fabric in the oil and take it with you when you go out – it can be tied around your neck, wrist or ankle or simply placed in a pocket.

A few drops of diluted essential oil of lavender applied to a bite or sting is remarkably soothing. A mixture of diluted peppermint oil and basil oil rubbed over any exposed parts of the body is reputed to have a marked deterrent effect and, if a bite or sting does occur when covered with this mixture, the pain is often not so bad. Many flying insects, particularly mosquitoes, dislike the smell of garlic, and eating large amounts of it can prove an effective deterrent as it will be detected by them in your perspiration. Again, rubbing the cut edge of a garlic clove on the site of any mosquito bites will help reduce the swelling.

Various growing plants have deterrent effects on insects. Flies, for example, are said to be repelled by eau-de-cologne mint and most midges and mosquitoes are repelled by garlic and ginger plants.

Pets often house insects in their fur. A strip of cotton fabric that has been soaked in a few drops of essential oil of penny-royal diluted in a carrier oil can be attached to your pet's collar to deter the most persistent of fleas without harming the animal. A few juniper berries tied in muslin can be attached in the same way or fastened to furniture. Geraniums have a deterrent effect on pet lice and the essential oil is very useful if these are a problem.

INSOMNIA

There are a number of ways of helping people suffering with this annoying complaint. Too much pent-up physical energy may make the situation worse, so giving yourself a physical challenge during the day may well help. This can take the form of a 20-minute walk, some gardening, or anything that will fit into your schedule; it doesn't have to be an organised sport. Taking a walk when the sun is going down is a wonderful way of marking the transition between the active, working part of the day and the gentler energy of evening (it can also yield some wonderfully restful views of sunsets). Or strolling out in the moonlight, if it is safe to do so, is a calming way to end the day.

Carrying out a security check before going to bed will

help allay any anxieties. Making a point of checking the locks on doors and windows, that the cooker is turned off, etc. can all form part of a soothing and calming bedtime ritual. Keeping a pencil and paper by the bed so that any late-night thoughts can be recorded and saved for the morning is another technique that will allow your mind to let go and relax. Having a warm bath amid candlelight and a hot drink shortly before bedtime is pacifying and, if milk is tolerated, a sweet milky drink can be very comforting. You may find that spraying your face and neck with cool (not cold) water helps calm you too, and listening to some gentle instrumental music or tapes of natural sounds may encourage sleep.

It may also be worth instigating some form of relaxation plan – anything that can be done in bed, such as systematically relaxing each muscle in your body, silently repeating some form of prayer, or even counting sheep!

A lime-blossom bath is delicately soothing and will help ease away the cares of the day. Take 125g (4oz) of freshly picked lime blossoms – this is one time when there really is no dried alternative – and soak them in 4.5 litres (1 gallon) of cold water for 12 hours. Heat gently, then strain into a warm bath. Lie in the bath for about 20 minutes, enjoying the fragrance of the blossoms, before retiring to bed.

A cup of valerian or lemon balm tea taken earlier in the evening has been known to encourage sleep. Lettuce is another natural soporific, so lettuce sandwiches for supper may help too. Hop tea has a gentle sedative effect, and hop pillows have been used for centuries to encourage sleep. However, they are not recommended for hayfever sufferers, and some people are allergic to the dried hops so it is important to check first.

The essential oils of clary sage, which is deeply relaxing and enhances dream quality, sandalwood and marjoram (very warming and comforting) can all help create a restful atmosphere for sleep. Add a few drops of these or any other sedative essential oils (lavender, chamomile, neroli, basil, etc.) to an oil burner or sprinkle them on to your pillow before retiring. Two drops may also be added to the bathwater to further boost its relaxing effect, or to a carrier oil for a massage. If there is somebody who will give you a massage before bed, this can be a truly wonderful way to end the day and prepare you for sleep. Self massage of the face and feet is a good alternative. Make gentle, circular movements at a very slow pace, paying particular attention to the forehead and temple region and to the delicate point just between the heel and the arch of the foot. Continue for as long as feels pleasurable. You could also make slow, gentle, sunwise circles on your abdomen, starting around the navel and making the circles larger and larger until much of the torso is covered. This is a very soothing and healing exercise. Any area of the body that you can reach will enjoy being massaged, and taking the time to relax yourself in this way will pay dividends.

Reading a really boring book on a subject of absolutely no interest to you usually works rather well, and more so if you have to get out of bed and turn on the lights to do so. On a more stimulating note, sex is a wonderful way to end the day and usually promotes deep, restful sleep.

If getting to sleep is imperative, prepare two cups of strong black coffee and two of chamomile tea. Once in bed, sip half a cup of coffee then half a cup of chamomile tea, followed by another half of coffee then another half of tea. This seems to win by confusing your body so much that it simply conks out. A drastic measure, and one that should not be repeated more than once a week, but it does work remarkably quickly – rarely are both drinks finished!

LARYNGITIS

We most often associate this condition with a lost voice, or with the deep, husky voice that often accompanies a cold. The one remedy that never seems to fail is to wrap the whole throat and neck overnight in a lard bandage.

Heat 1kg (2lb) of lard gently in a saucepan until it melts and then soak a strip of clean cotton fabric in it. Stir the cotton around, making sure that it is thoroughly coated with the lard. Meanwhile, smear a drop or two of pure unroasted sesame oil around the neck, allowing a little to cover the chin and the top of the shoulders as well. Once the cotton strip is cool enough to handle, wrap it once around the neck. Cover quickly with an old towel and place another towel around the shoulders in case of drips.

This can be left in place overnight and is surprisingly comfortable and comforting. The wrap can be repeated every second night and it is rarely needed more than twice.

Laryngitis can be seen as a wonderful opportunity to rest the voice, particularly if you have been overusing it. The best general advice is to allow your body to take its own course, making sure that you have plenty of rest, fresh air and relaxation, until you are ready to begin communicating once again.

MENOPAUSE

This is such a key time in every woman's life that I would strongly recommend working with a naturopath or natural healthcare practitioner, who will be able to help make this transition as smooth and problem-free as possible. It is also a time of great change on the emotional and psychological levels, and a good relationship with a practitioner can provide valuable support and encouragement. Some women sail through the menopause smoothly without any upset or discomfort, while others may experience a whole range of symptoms. Since each woman's experience is different, the individual care a practitioner can offer is invaluable in tailoring whatever treatment may be required.

A number of dietary changes will help minimise mood swings and energy fluctuations, and switching to a hypoglycaemic diet will have instant positive effects. Very simply, this means maintaining constant blood sugar levels by eating every four hours and increasing the unrefined carbohydrate content of each meal. Taking hot and cold showers (always finish with cold) and barefoot walks in the early morning dew will help stimulate the system and keep the whole body working at an optimum.

Yarrow hip baths taken every other day are one of the most effective overall measures to reduce symptoms and improve energy levels. Take 125g (4oz) of yarrow and place it in a large container. Cover with 4.5 litres (1 gallon) of cold water and leave to stand for 12 hours. Heat the mixture gently and then just as it reaches boiling point strain the liquid into a hot bath. This needs to be full enough to cover the kidney area of the mid back. Stay in the bath for about 20 minutes, then wrap up well and go and lie down for at least two hours.

Taking regular weight-bearing exercise is an important measure to help guard against osteoporosis, the bone thinning that responds to hormonal changes and increases after the menopause. The simplest form of weight-bearing exercise is walking, which can offer great benefits at any time of life but especially now.

Hormone replacement therapy (HRT) is currently gaining in popularity but it is worth noting that there is a huge variety of herbal remedies and compounds that will stimulate or simulate hormonal action without any debilitating side effects. Lady's mantle is just one of a number of herbs that may be taken regularly as a tea throughout a woman's life and it has a very positive effect on the system during menopause. The herb *Mitchella repens* is also a tremendously effective 'women's herb', and its common name, squaw vine, reflects that, although this name is now being dropped as people realise the offensive connotations of the word squaw. This herb was introduced to foreign settlers by Native American Indian women. Other oestrogen-rich herbs include blessed thistle and false unicorn root. Liquorice is also an oestrogen derivative, and fennel tea, one of the more pleasant-tasting teas, contains valuable plant oestrogens. Foods rich in oestrogen include sprouted seeds, bananas and whole grains so it is important to include large amounts of these in the diet. Vitamin E stimulates oestrogen production, and a supplement of up to 1,000 iu a day will be helpful.

A daily cup of sage tea will give you an overall lift – be sure to sip it slowly and finish it while it is still warm. Lemon balm leaves may be added to salads or made into a tea for their calming effect – drink up to three cups a day. One cup of tansy tea taken in the early evening, or one very weak cup of pennyroyal (never exceed one cup per day, and only take it if you are experiencing night sweats as part of the menopause) may help reduce night sweats, but my favourite remedy for this is essential oil of clary sage. Add two drops to a little carrier oil and gently massage it into the wrists, hands and face, paying particular attention to the temples. Doing this before bedtime will make a real difference, and this herb has the added benefit of making sleep easier and enhancing dreams.

Essential oils of rose and geranium can be used to great effect to support other measures. Geranium is a hormonal balancer, while rose tones and cleanses the uterus, helps stabilise the menstrual cycle, and nurtures the emotional, feminine side. This may be an important benefit if there is any question of femininity being somehow 'lost' or self-esteem being at a low ebb. A few drops of either oil may be added to the bathwater, used in an oil burner or sprinkled on to a pillow or handkerchief.

MENSTRUAL DIFFICULTIES

Painful periods are so common that my patients often have to be prompted to mention them as a complaint, accepting them as a matter of course. This is quite simply not true. If it hurts, it is because something is wrong. The doctors that my patients have encountered (women as well as men) appear to believe that pain in the body indicates a problem UNLESS it is related to menstruation, in which case it is quite normal. I have heard of women who faint each month because of the pain from their periods and yet they are told that this is quite normal. Bunkum.

Neither is it normal to function competently for four or five days each month only through the effects of strong pain killers.

If periods are always painful, please consult a naturopath or natural healthcare practitioner who will help you do something about it. If your current practitioner won't, then change to another practitioner.

The symptoms can be helped in a number of natural ways. Many women find dramatic relief from a range of difficulties simply by switching from tampons to external protection. Herbs, a traditional 'women's way', come into their own for treating menstrual conditions. Equal parts of dried lady's mantle and dried yarrow make a wonderfully effective tea that can be taken once a day. Cover the herbs with boiling water, leave to stand for about 30 seconds, then strain. Sip the tea slowly, making sure to finish it before it is completely cold. This tea eases period pains and can be taken daily, starting six to seven days before your period is due and stopping when it arrives. It will also help make your cycle regular so it is useful when periods are absent, scanty or irregular. One cup each day of the water in which French beans have been boiled will also help cleanse the pelvic area.

Including large amounts of onions and raw parsley in your diet will help regulate the cycle and have a clearing, cleansing effect. The tissue salts Mag. Phos. and Nat. Mur can both help with regulating the cycle and reducing premenstrual tension and water retention. Taking 0.3ml of freshly prepared tincture of myrrh (if tolerated) twice a day, will have a regulating effect on water balance very quickly. The homoeopathic remedy Rhus. Tox. may relieve the pain, and supplementing it with the mineral silica may help regulate any menstrual abnormalities. These both have a long-term effect, and best results will be seen after a few months.

Far and away the most effective treatment I have encountered is to fast or follow a raw diet for three days at the time of ovulation. Start the diet ten days after the first day's bleeding of your last period. This seems to reduce problems when your period arrives. In cold weather a three-day brown rice and beetroot diet or grape mono-diet seems to work better than a completely raw diet, which is best for the spring, summer and warmer autumn days. During either, drinking large amounts of hot water to which a sliver of fresh ginger root has been added will help keep the body feeling warm.

Massage around the navel is very soothing, can help relieve

pain and will also encourage the flow if periods are irregular. Using your thumb or your middle three fingers held closely together, massage the area around the navel, using very slow, quite deep, circular movements. Don't be afraid to press deeply; as long as you move slowly the feeling should be extremely pleasant and give great relief if pain is present. Complete a number of circles around the navel and then make bigger and bigger circles using a progressively lighter pressure, but remaining slow and careful until much of the abdomen is being covered. You will be able to gauge the amount of pressure that feels good. As a general rule, the area closest to the navel can take a firm pressure, so long as it is applied slowly and carefully, and the pressure needs to be lighter the further away you are from this point.

A number of essential oils can also help at this time. Adding a few drops of lavender and geranium to a base of almond, soya or pure unroasted sesame oil for massaging around the navel will enhance the soothing effect. Burning howood oil in an oil burner will reduce pelvic congestion, while a few drops of clary sage added to a burner or used in dilution in a massage oil will have a positive overall effect. This oil is best used at bedtime or during a period of relaxation and should not be used before driving or operating any machinery.

There is a variety of useful exercises and postures, particularly those which tilt the angle of the womb. The simplest of these is to lie on a slant board (see page 18). Otherwise, get on your hands and knees and bend your elbows so that your chest falls slowly towards the floor. Turning your head to one side, you can release your arms and let them lie wherever they are most comfortable. Essentially what you are doing is sticking your bottom up in the air, and the longer you stay in this position the longer you are likely to be pain-free afterwards. You should experience relief quite quickly so staying there is no hardship. You might also experiment with tilting the angle of the pelvis in other ways – by propping it up on cushions when you lie down or adjusting the angle of your chair.

Making a sandwich of the pelvis between two hot-water

bottles and keeping that entire area warm and well covered will help steady the flow of blood and bring comfort. Walking is a good, gentle exercise for alleviating period pains, as is any soft, rhythmic action you can make with the pelvis. Sex is a wonderful aid to periods – regular orgasms help tone the pelvic muscles and regulate the cycle. The release of energy in this way may also relieve pre-menstrual tension.

Our attitude to menstruation is very important. While it is still regarded as a negative thing – painful, somewhat dirty or shameful, and certainly not a topic for polite conversation – it is little wonder if it is an unpleasant or difficult event. This time could be a regular celebration of our connectedness with nature and the life cycle; a time of rejoicing in heightened intuition and increased personal power; a time to retreat into one's inner depths for regeneration and renewal; a time of receiving for ourselves rather than continually being the source for others. Any form of ritual that reinforces this positive aspect, from having a massage to entering a silent retreat, will help ensure that menstruation is a positive, joyful time both physically and emotionally.

MIGRAINE

I have a particular interest in this condition because it is what prompted me to investigate natural healthcare in the first place. During my late teens and early twenties I suffered with terrible migraines that would appear without any warning and last for two to three days. During that time I was completely unable to do anything. The pain was so intolerable that I could not eat and could barely drink or move from my bed. On a few occasions I lost the ability to speak as well. These frightening attacks began recurring more and more frequently until I was experiencing at least one a month.

Although my GP was sympathetic, the only treatment he could offer was some tablets which I had to take every single day and which, he said, might not even help at all. The only positive result of this was that it spurred me on to consult a naturopath who used dietary therapy, osteopathy, a few herbs and some acupuncture, and within a couple of months my whole system felt totally different. The migraines became less and less frequent and a range of other minor health complaints disappeared too.

The measures outlined below may sound quite stringent but if you suffer with migraines I know you will be prepared to try them. Do not follow them for more than two months without seeking the advice of a naturopath or natural health-care practitioner.

There is a tendency nowadays to call any painful headache a migraine. What differentiates these attacks is that they often include nausea and acute aversion to any source of light. Movement is extremely difficult, and the pain in the head is often intense and pulsating and most usually one sided. Some people may have a warning up to a few hours before the onset of the greatest pain; this can take the form of a range of visual disturbances, including temporary one-sided blindness and blurred vision.

The first thing to do is look at your diet. Many people find they have an intolerance to particular foods, the main culprits being chocolate, cheese and red wine. Once the liver is working better and the migraines have begun to disappear these foods can be reintroduced, but until then they should be strictly avoided. I would also recommend avoiding all types of alcohol (although sherry and port seem to be the worst), coffee, oranges, tomatoes, spinach, sorrel and rhubarb. Often with migraines the gall bladder is underfunctioning, (along with the liver) so reduce the amount of fat you eat and look out for hidden fats in foods such as ice cream. Avoid hydrogenated fats and oils completely.

Keeping a diet diary (see page 23) is the best way to isolate any foods that may be causing the migraine. Record your feelings as well as the foods you eat, and keep a note of when your migraines appear. Over four to six weeks a pattern should begin to emerge. Eating regularly so that your blood sugar levels do not drop, and taking care not to over-exert yourself, will also help keep your body in balance.

The herb feverfew will grow just about anywhere and is

well worth cultivating because one cup a day of an infusion made with a few fresh leaves will often be enough to stave off regular attacks. It can also be taken at the very beginning of a migraine and, if caught early enough, it may abort the attack. Feverfew leaves may also be chewed at the onset of an attack, or taken that way on a regular basis in preference to the tea.

Placing cool compresses (see page 5) on your forehead and the back of your neck may help with the pounding pain. Some people suggest using essential oil of lavender but I find that the sense of smell is so heightened during an attack that even the pleasing scent of lavender can become offensive. So if in doubt, do without.

A hot compress (see page 5) placed over the liver will bring gradual relief in some cases, although I prefer to use it as a nightly preparation during the interval between attacks.

It is important to feel some sense of control, and imagining your hands becoming cooler and warmer by turn seems to be the most effective form of visualisation. This also helps regulate the passage of blood through the neck region. As congestion in this area can be a major cause of migraines, this is a doubly effective technique.

If you combine all these measures with a thorough osteopathic check up, where the condition of the neck and lower back will be investigated and, if necessary, treated, they may put an end to your migraine headaches.

Menstruation and ovulation can influence women's sensitivity to migraine triggers (see **Menstrual Difficulties**). Curiously, most migraines that are due to or aggravated by food intolerance tend to disappear after the third month of pregnancy. Although they often reappear at some time after giving birth, this does make a welcome break from dietary restrictions.

NAUSEA

Nausea can have all sorts of causes. It is a normal reaction when the body needs to rid itself of something, and it can also occur in response to upsets such as travelling or overheating. Persistent nausea may be a sign that the body needs to expel toxins, and some form of elimination or detox diet would be recommended. See page 20 for a simple cleansing diet, and consider visiting your naturopath or natural healthcare practitioner for a full diagnosis and advice on cleansing your system. In the meantime, increase the amount of good, clean water you drink to flush the system, and maintain blood sugar levels by eating regular meals and avoiding sugar and refined foods. It is helpful to avoid stimulants such as caffeine and to eat foods rich in B vitamins or take a supplement of 500mg B complex each day.

An immediate way to settle the stomach is to chew a piece of crystallised ginger very slowly. This has a particularly beneficial effect if vomiting has already occurred or if there is any related gastrointestinal upset. Simply drinking some warm water will settle the stomach in most cases and also soothe and calm the body generally.

Nausea can be the body's way of saying that it needs more air, a message that can be easily attended to. If the waves of nausea are fairly mild, eating a piece of dry wholemeal toast or a cracker may help. More settling for the system, though, is a cup of liquorice root tea, or a special Ayurvedic blend of tea called Vata which is especially soothing.

NEURALGIA

This is a severe stabbing pain which can be felt along the course of the facial nerves. It may be due to injury, exposure to cold and draughts, dental work, or many other causes.

One of the nicest cures is gently rubbing the juice of an organically grown lemon over the skin of the entire affected area. This is cooling, acts as a nerve tonic and has anti-inflammatory properties. If repeated once an hour relief should be gained within half a day. A few drops of essential oil of lemon can also be added to an oil burner or to a vase of warm water placed near a radiator or other heat source. This continues the positive effect of the treatment in between applications. Note that essential oil of lemon should not be applied to the skin.

Alternatively, make a strong tea with fresh verbena leaves, soak a cotton wool pad in the liquid and apply it to the site of the pain, using light pressure. Repeat once the first compress has cooled and then every hour until relief is apparent. Witch hazel may be heated and used in the same way and has a lightly astringent effect on the skin, which may help with localised sensitivity.

The sort of treatment offered by a cranial osteopath or cranio-sacral therapist (see page 12) can be very effective, and in some cases relief can be instantaneous.

NOSEBLEEDS

There must be almost as many home cures for nosebleeds as there are for hiccoughs! If they are a frequent problem, make sure you consume plenty of vitamin C. The easiest way to achieve this is by eating five portions of fresh fruit and vegetables each day. A vitamin C supplement of up to 3g a day should make an immediate difference. If nosebleeds are occurring regularly, consult your naturopath or natural healthcare practitioner.

The strangest yet one of the most effective remedies I know is to wind a rubber band quite tightly around each little finger, at the tip near the nail. This seems to work within a matter of minutes. Once the rubber bands have been removed the bleeding will not usually start again. Another old remedy is to place a cold wet towel on the back between the shoulder blades and then lie down. The dropping of a cold key down the back of the sufferer's shirt or dress is, I suppose, a modern equivalent.

Although it shouldn't really work – there is no anatomical reason for it – applying pressure to the point of the nose where the hard bone ends and the softer tissue begins often stops bleeding dramatically quickly. This area can then be covered with a cold compress (see page 5) to retain the benefit.

OEDEMA

Oedema, or swelling, may be the body's way of immobilising an area in order to keep it safe or a sign that the body's own self-regulating mechanisms cannot quite cope. A classic example of swelling to immobilise or splint the area is as a reaction to some form of injury, when movement would put additional strain on a damaged structure. The second type of swelling is often seen during pregnancy, when the legs and ankles in particular may become slightly swollen because of the extra weight that the abdomen is having to deal with.

Both cases respond to the same type of treatment. Applying cold water is the first step towards encouraging a fresh blood supply to the area. This not only brings in fresh nutrients to help with any necessary repair work but also increases the action of the lymphatic system in removing any unnecessary build-up from the area. If possible, the affected area can simply be held under the cold tap for five minutes. Otherwise, a piece of cotton fabric can be soaked in cold water, wrung out and applied to the area, repeating as often as possible to ensure that it remains cold. If the swollen area has been caused by an injury and is very small, ice can be applied instead of cold water (see **Sprains**).

The next step is to make it easier for the body to achieve the increased circulation that will be required after the hydrotherapy treatment. This can best be done by raising the swollen area above the level of the heart for as long as possible. If the legs are affected the easiest way to do this is to raise the foot of the bed at night by placing a few telephone directories underneath it.

If the oedema is generalised and there is water retention throughout the body, then one cup of dandelion tea each day will make a difference. Hot ginger compresses (see page 5) applied to the kidneys once a day will also start to get things moving. It is most important to reduce the amount of salt in the diet and the tissue salt Nat. Mur. is a good support while trying to achieve this. Instead of salt use a variety of herbs to season your food. Fresh chamomile, juniper berries, marshmallow flowers, ginger root and parsley will all assist in cleansing the body, as well as drawing the taste buds away from their desire for salt.

OPERATION AND OTHER SCARS

Small wounds will be much less likely to result in scarring if they are packed with a bunch of fresh common thyme. Otherwise, Swedish bitters applied regularly to the scar will reduce it considerably. This old recipe of herbs, plants and roots was formulated by a Dr Samst, who claimed that only 40 applications were necessary to make a scar all but disappear.

Operation wounds heal more quickly if calendula ointment is applied every day. Cranio-sacral therapy (see page 12) can also be very effective at this time. It offers a specific technique for working with the fascia (the connective tissue that wraps around every muscle and organ in the body like a sort of natural clingfilm), which is necessarily cut through or otherwise disturbed during an operation. Settling it and relieving any associated tensions through cranial treatment will accelerate healing.

PILES

See **Haemorrhoids**.

POOR CIRCULATION

Many people suffer with poor circulation, particularly towards the end of the winter months when the body's resources appear to be running low. It can seem as if the effort of keeping warm, against nature's efforts to freeze everything in the world, is starting to prove too big a job.

Surprisingly, one of the most effective remedies for constantly cold hands and feet is cold-water paddling. Each morning before bathing or showering, fill the bath or a washing-up bowl with enough cold water to cover the ankles and walk up and down or walk on the spot for at least 120 steps. Plunging the feet into cold water in this way seems to appeal directly to the most primitive level of our physical awareness. The body rapidly sends the feet a fresh, warming, nutrient-rich supply of blood and this increase in circulation warms not just the feet but the entire body for quite some time. People usually find that by the time they step out of the water their feet are glowingly warm and remain that way for much of the rest of the day.

Adding a small amount of cayenne pepper to at least one meal each day will have a stimulating effect on the circulatory system, and you can also sprinkle a little in your socks or stockings. It has a tendency to colour your toes but really does improve circulation.

Ginger is another worthwhile addition to the diet. A small piece the size of a fingertip, peeled and chopped or pushed through a garlic press and added to any meal at the cooking stage, can make a big difference. Or the ginger can be placed whole in a cup and covered with boiling water for a surprisingly pleasant-tasting tea. This stimulates the appetite as well, so is a useful thing to drink in the winter months before the main meal of the day.

If you have become chilled or your feet have turned numb from standing in the cold, a hot mustard foot bath is the best possible all-round tonic (see page 16). This also makes for an excellent measure if trying to stave off a cold.

PRURITIS

Really this just means itching, but it is generally used to refer to itching in the genital area. An itching bottom will respond well to stimulation of a corresponding energy point on the meridian system of the body. Draw an imaginary line from the top of each ear straight up to the crown of the head so that you reach a point in the middle of the scalp. Gentle, slow and deep circular massage of this point will stop itching and also help prevent soreness and piles. It works within minutes and can be repeated as often as the itch occurs. I feel it is best to massage in a sunwise circle, but if the opposite way feels better then do that.

If the bottom itches only at night, check for worms. The easiest way to do this is to stick a small strip of adhesive tape over the anus before going to sleep. If worms are responsible for the itching, the evidence will be there on the tape in the morning. Any infestation like this is best treated with the aid of a naturopath or natural healthcare practitioner but cutting down on sugar and yeast (see page 74) and eating more fresh garlic are good general rules that should make a difference quite quickly.

Genital itching associated with thrush will respond well to regular bathing in warm water to which has been added five drops of tincture of myrrh (see **Thrush**).

Tight-fitting clothing made of synthetic fibres will only exacerbate this condition, so switch to cotton underwear (or none at all whenever possible) and wear stockings instead of tights.

PSORIASIS

This chronic skin disorder can be extremely painful and distressing. The condition of the skin is a reflection of internal health, and psoriasis is often associated with thinning of the bowel wall. Diet, therefore, is the first approach when trying to shift this stubborn condition.

Psoriasis sufferers often have difficulty digesting saturated fats, in addition to a variety of other difficulties such as underfunction of the liver and kidneys. Because of this an excess of animal products in the diet can prove highly aggravating. Poor elimination is also a common problem and one of the most effective ways of treating this is prolonged fasting and vegetable juice mono-diets. These should only be undertaken with the advice and support of a naturopath or natural healthcare practitioner.

As well as animal products, exclude citrus fruits, hydrogenated fats, wheat, yeast, sugar and refined foods from your diet and you should see an improvement in your condition. Specific foods to add to your diet include sea vegetables, olive oil (about one tablespoon a day) and at least one meal of raw salad daily. Supplements of 3g daily of vitamin C with bioflavonoids and vitamin E, beginning with 100iu each day and increasing the amount every three days to about 1000iu, plus a minimum dose of 500iu of vitamin A will all help.

Regular bowel movements are absolutely essential, and care must be taken to ensure that none of the eliminative channels becomes impaired. Applying a castor oil pack to the abdomen each evening is particularly soothing and will help ensure a bowel movement the following morning.

Castor Oil Pack

SOAK a large piece of plain undyed wool in castor oil and place it in a saucepan. Heat it gently, then fold it and lay it on the right side of the abdomen, covering it from the lowest rib right down to the top of the pubic bone. It should be as hot as you can bear and needs to remain in place for at least 45 minutes and up to 90 minutes. To hold the heat in, cover the pack with a plastic bag and place a hot-water bottle on top, or wrap with blankets or a duvet. After removing the pack, wash the skin with warm water to which has been added a large pinch of bicarbonate of soda (about 1 teaspoon to 1.2 litres (2 pints) of water).

Good bowel health will make the job of the liver easier, helping to speed up the process of detoxifying the body. To support this, drink a glass of fresh raw beetroot juice every day or eat a portion of fresh raw beetroot, and drink a cup of dandelion coffee. Dandelion coffee may be drunk freely as a coffee substitute, but limit the amount of milk you add and if you want to sweeten it, use honey. A supplement of the herb silymarine (milk thistle) may also be taken to support the liver – begin with the minimum dose recommended on the packet and take it for three days, then have one day off. Repeat this for two weeks, and then progress to the regular recommended dose.

Taking 10ml fresh cleavers juice each day along with one cup of strong red clover tea will help by reducing cell production. Psoriasis means that some skin cells are over-produced yet fail to mature into normal keratin. The cleavers/red clover combination should delay this effect for long enough for other measures such as the bowel cleansing to take hold.

All activities that boost the lymphatic system will show good results. Cold-water paddling (see **Poor Circulation**), air baths (see **Body Odour**) sunbathing and dry skin brushing (see page 17) all help enormously and should be performed as regularly as possible. Adding a capful of apple cider vinegar to the bathwater and avoiding soap will assist the pH balance of the skin. An alternative cleansing agent which is also very soothing and has great therapeutic value is a handful of oatmeal and a pinch of marshmallow root, wrapped in a cotton handkerchief and then tied to the hot water tap while the bath is running. Allow the bag to sit in the bath with you, and enjoy.

Fresh plantain leaves can be applied directly to more stubborn skin lesions and are enormously soothing. If these are not available, plantain oil may be used instead. Another application is pure unroasted sesame oil blended with a few drops of fresh celandine or mallow juice. This may be used to cover large areas of skin and is both soothing and healing.

RHEUMATISM

See **Arthritis**.

RINGWORM

This is a fungal condition that appears as discrete round patches of raised and reddened skin and is remarkably itchy.

Removing all sugar and yeast from the diet, including mushrooms and mycoproteins, will help correct any internal imbalance (see page 74). The fungus thrives in warm, moist conditions, so keeping the body cool will help with the itching and soreness, and drinking peppermint tea (hot or cold) will help cool the body down. The tea may also be used as a wash for the affected areas, or the teabag or herb itself used as a cold compress (see page 5). This is very soothing and shows good results quite quickly.

Cover each of the affected areas with set honey as many times each day as possible. If applied often enough this starves the site of oxygen and heals the area. Leave uncovered once the honey has been applied, and be sure to apply a thick covering before going to bed. This does mean sticky bedcovers for a few nights but the honey cure is so effective that it is well worth it.

SHINGLES

See **Herpes**.

SHOCK

Shock can cause untold difficulties because it is a way of reacting to events or injury by retreating deep into ourselves and withdrawing our energy from part or most of the body.

By far the best initial treatment for shock is to have somebody hold you. A long, warm hug from someone who cares will help you keep the feeling of remaining in your body. Their physical warmth and emotional help are both equally important.

If you are alone, breathing into the area that has been hurt or, if it is a more general thing, then breathing into your main energy centre just below the navel will have a similar effect. It is helpful to reinforce this with the touch of another person as soon as possible. In the meantime, close your eyes and feel your breath and the energy of life that it contains reaching down into the centre of your body, warming as it goes. Breathe deeply, taking in as much life force as you can muster with each breath, draw it right down into the belly, then relax and enjoy the full, warm feeling as your body automatically exhales. Keep this up for as long as it takes for you to feel calm and settled.

Dr Bach's Rescue Remedy is an excellent remedy for shock and can be taken on its own or in a little water. Since it contains alcohol, you may prefer to rub it on to the pulse points in your wrists and neck. If you have had an accident requiring hospital treatment it is important to inform the medical staff that the remedy has been used in this way – if there is a suspicion of drunkenness because of the smell of alcohol this may well affect treatment options.

After any incidence of shock it is well worth spending some time going over the event with someone you feel you can talk to freely. This might be a friend or relative or a counsellor or other practitioner. Try to get rid of any associated feelings and worries so that you can recover from the whole affair, and maybe even learn from it.

Shock and stresses generally place enormous strain on the kidneys, so a cup of goldenrod tea can be a tremendous aid. Steep a heaped tablespoon of goldenrod in a mug of boiling water for about 30 seconds, then remove. The hot tea should be sipped slowly, and up to three cups a day can be taken. It has quite a delicious, saffron-type flavour, but if you prefer you may add a little sweetener.

SINUS COMPLAINTS

Sinus congestion is not just caused by colds and flu; it may also be the result of allergies or a build-up of mucus, or the sinuses may be a weak spot. The pain and headaches resulting from blocked sinuses can be really debilitating and sometimes the chest may become congested too.

The sinuses are spaces within the skull, and one of their jobs is to give resonance to the voice. They are lined with mucous membrane in the same way as the throat. The ones most commonly affected are those just above the brow and below the eye. When the body produces excess mucus these spaces can quickly fill up and their small drainage holes become incapable of removing the excess material.

On another level, sinus congestion can often be an indicator of a need to cry, and weeping does tend to relieve the sinuses more effectively than anything else. I was brought up to believe in the magical powers of salt water, and releasing pent-up tears does seem to bear out the truth of this.

The first step in managing any sinus condition is to reduce the amount of mucus produced by the body. Diet plays an important role here, and eliminating mucus-forming foods can have dramatic and immediate results. Following the three-day cleansing diet on page 20 will help your body to rally its resources and concentrate on healing itself.

This is also a good opportunity to take a look at your general eating habits in case the sinus congestion is caused by allergies. One of the most common allergies is to cow's products, so an over-reliance on these foods may be at the root of the difficulty (see **Allergies**).

A pinch of turmeric added to each meal during cooking will help reduce mucus congestion. This lovely yellow spice is both a liver stimulant and a useful way of reducing phlegm anywhere in the body. Chilli has a similar effect, so any hot and spicy meals will help at this time.

An old-fashioned steam inhalation can be very effective in clearing the sinuses. Pour boiled water into a bowl and then bend over it and cover your head and the bowl with a towel.

Breathing in the steam through the nose and the mouth will help clear the congestion. Herbs will speed up the process and they have their own therapeutic effects: a sprig of rosemary added to the water has antiseptic qualities, and thyme and sage have a soothing effect.

A few drops of essential oil can also be used: rosemary, if you don't have the fresh herb; eucalyptus if there is any accompanying chest congestion; or Olbas Oil, which will cut through the most stubbornly blocked sinuses. These essential oils may also be added to a light carrier oil such as almond, soya or pure unroasted sesame, and used to massage the face and neck gently. A gentle massage technique called tapotment is best used around the eyes and across the cheek bones – anywhere you can feel the bone immediately underneath the skin. To do this, place your middle finger over your index finger so that the middle fingertip weighs upon the index fingertip and tap with a light, springing action all around the eyes. Go slowly at first and take great care to avoid the eye. This percussive movement will soon loosen any mucus congestion and give great relief.

You could also try draining the under-eye sinus by lying with your head on one side and stroking fairly firmly along the cheekbone towards the nose. Do this first on one side, then the other. Keep a handkerchief handy but try not to blow hard, rather just mop up any runniness.

Finish any facial massage with gentle strokes down the cheek muscles from just in front of each ear to the angle of the jaw, and take some long, firm, sweeping strokes down the back of the neck towards the lymph nodes. This will help drain the lymphatic system.

SPRAINS

A sprain occurs when the ligaments surrounding a joint are unduly stretched (usually suddenly) or torn completely. Normally, muscles help protect the joints and prevent the ligaments being harmed. During an unexpected movement, or when pushing the joint beyond its normal range of movement, the muscles may be caught unawares and the ligaments will end up taking the full force of the strain.

Wherever the site of the sprain, the treatment is always the same. RICE is the keyword:

Rest
Ice
Compression
Elevation

Rest is rather obvious. Stop whatever you are doing and ensure that no more weight or strain is put on the affected joint. Sprains are often acutely painful and the pain wears off slowly, so you will probably be only too eager to rest, but if you are tempted to try and carry on through the pain, remember this may cause further damage to the joint.

Ice is the next step. Apply an ice pack to the joint as soon as you possibly can to help reduce any swelling (see **Backache**). The body has an incredibly fast response to accidents such as this and will seek to immobilise the area as fast as it can by causing it to swell; it is your job to get there with the ice first. The cold will encourage a good supply of blood and nutrients to the area and will stimulate the lymphatic system into carrying away any damaged cells and other debris. Ice will also reduce bleeding from torn blood vessels and help minimise the pain – an important consideration. Keep the ice pack in place for 30 minutes, then remove and repeat for 15 minutes at a time with 10-minute breaks.

Compression is next. Bandage or strap the affected joint if you know how. Otherwise, wrap the ice pack quite tightly around the joint with yet another tea-towel or a scarf. This measure prevents further swelling and, depending on the severity of the pain, you can choose to use a straight bandage, which can be left in place for 24 hours, or an ice pack which will need to be replaced often. Make sure you wrap only the joint and not the surrounding area.

Elevation last of all, but equally important. Raise the affected limb and support it well to enable blood to flow towards the heart. This reduces the pressure of fluid on the injured area. Ideally the limb should be rested above the level of the heart, so lying down is a good idea, but if this is not possible then simply supporting it – for example, putting an injured leg on a cushion-covered chair or stool – will suffice.

RICE is easy to remember and easy to apply. Putting it into practice as soon as possible after an injury occurs is the best way to minimise pain and maximise healing. The homoeopathic remedy arnica should also be taken once the RICE procedure has been instigated.

Bioflavonoids are food for the collagen fibres of the body and, together with vitamin C which speeds recovery from injuries, they should be taken in doses of up to 1g of vitamin C with bioflavonoids every hour for up to three hours after the sprain. They can be continued at the lower dose of twice a day.

Vitamins A and E and zinc may also be taken in a multi-vitamin and mineral formula immediately after the injury. Vitamin A promotes wound healing; vitamin E reinforces this and helps control the inflammation; while zinc helps in both these processes.

Turmeric is a very useful aid in inflammatory conditions. It can be taken internally by sprinkling it on meals or using it in cooking, or it can be made into a poultice (see page 6) by mixing it with slaked lime (available from health-food shops and some chemists). This ancient remedy has a good effect if there is an old injury but also works speedily to reduce inflammation if the sprain is a recent one.

I remember spraining my ankle once when I was a child. The shooting pain was relieved within minutes when my father lovingly worked all around the joint with warm, careful movements. The massage was part of the cure but the loving contact meant a lot too. Whenever we injure ourselves, even slightly, there is a sense of shock, and of our energy withdrawing from the affected area (see **Shock**). The physical touch of a healer or someone who cares can allow us to relax back into our body and begin to repair the damage. Gentle self-massage can also be very helpful, and may be done as soon as you feel able. Work slowly and quite deeply all around the affected area, using just enough pressure so that it feels good – there is a point at which you may feel some discomfort but it should seem like a good contact, rather like scratching a deep itch. Finish the massage with some passive mobilisations – this means taking the joint slowly and carefully through its full range of movement without using the muscles. If you let your hand relax completely and go limp and heavy, and then move it around with your other hand, you'll be practising passive movements.

If the injury is bad then specialist remedial massage may be necessary and you can find this at a sports injury clinic or similar, but with minor sprains home treatment will be fine.

STYES

These unsightly and itchy bumps on the edge of the eyelid can be caused by bacteria, and quick treatment helps prevent them spreading.

The old country remedy was to rub the stye with a piece of gold, and this can still be effective. More modern methods include washing the eye with a mixture of eyebright and burdock tinctures (two drops of each tincture in a small tumbler of water) and ensuring that the main eliminative routes are working well. It is surprising how many styes, and lumps and bumps generally, occur because of a congested bowel (see **Constipation**).

Rubbing the stye with the cut edge of a piece of fresh marshmallow root will relieve the itchiness.

SUNBURN

The potential hazards of sunbathing are becoming better known and, thankfully, sunburn is now seen less often than even five years ago. With the damage that is still being done to our ozone layer, the potential for burning is present throughout the summer months and increasingly so at other times of year. Those of us in more temperate climates used to feel safe in gentle spring sunshine or on late autumn days, but this is no longer the case, and protection is a must whenever there is exposure to the sun.

If sunstroke is suspected, seek medical help immediately. Cold wet compresses applied to the back of the neck and the forehead (see page 5) should help while assistance is found. The addition of two drops of essential oil of lavender will calm and soothe the sufferer, and two drops of essential oil of lemongrass will help bring them round it fainting is a possibility.

Sunburn can be treated using any of the measures outlined for **Burns**. Particular attention must be paid to replacing any fluid loss, so take frequent drinks of water or heavily diluted fruit juice.

If you have an aloe plant, split open a leaf and apply the thick soothing gel over the affected area. Aloe juice (available in cartons) may also be sprayed on to the whole body at regular intervals (up to five times a day) and is particularly soothing if kept refrigerated.

Vinegar Wash

A VINEGAR wash is an excellent measure for sunburn, soothing almost immediately. I first encountered it while on holiday in Gibraltar.

Stir a cup of apple cider vinegar (you can use malt vinegar if apple cider is not available) into a bowl of tepid water and sponge any affected areas or the whole body with the solution. Squeeze the sponge lightly, just above the skin, so that no pressure is used on the skin itself and the liquid can gently run over the body. this is best applied as soon as sunburn is noticed, but will have a good effect at any time.

For small patches of sunburn, such as on the face or feet, an old German folk remedy is to put a couple of tomatoes in the fridge until they are quite cold, then slice them thinly and place on the burned area. It's odd, but it works.

SUNSTROKE

See **Sunburn**.

THRUSH

This candida fungus overgrowth may affect the mouth, skin or nails, yet most commonly occurs in and around the vagina. The symptoms of burning, irritation, constant itchiness and heavy, creamy discharge can cause great discomfort and distress.

Many women notice a connection between taking antibiotics and developing vaginal thrush; in fact some doctors now prescribe anti-thrush medication with certain antibiotics. Antibiotics work by killing bacteria and they kill all sorts of beneficial bacteria and micro-organisms as well as the problem ones. This means that the delicate balance of the body becomes disrupted even further, and problems occur in sites where this balance is crucial, such as the gut and the vagina.

Other factors that upset the pH balance of the vagina include a diet that is high in sugar and yeast, taking the contraceptive pill, and long-term stress. All these factors could apply to any number of women today. Some women may also find that they develop thrush as a localised reaction to some spermicidal creams and gels, and even to rubber.

Treatment needs to be both general, to deal with the fungal overgrowth and redress the body's pH levels, and localised, to help relieve the symptoms.

Dietary changes will boost energy levels and begin to have an effect quite quickly. It is important to eliminate all yeast products, including mushrooms and dishes made with mycoproteins, and all sugars from the diet (see page 74). Also avoid cow's dairy products, and wheat. Make sure to have at least six helpings of raw vegetables each day and one exclusively raw salad meal, if possible. Large amounts of garlic, onions and parsley can be added to the diet, the more the better. Garlic is a natural antibiotic which will help boost the body's defences without causing any side effects. All members of the onion family are great cleansers. Parsley has a high iron content and blood-enriching qualities and helps direct the cleansing towards the pelvic region.

It is also important to drink large amounts of fresh water, at least 1.5 litres (2½ pints) a day, and three glasses of unsweetened cranberry juice, spread throughout the day, to cleanse the urinary system. Avoid all stimulants such as caffeine, switch to herbal teas and plain hot water instead.

Apply liberal amounts of plain goat's or sheep's milk yoghurt (straight from the fridge for the best effect) to soothe local inflammation and relieve itching. The easiest way to do this is by placing one or two tablespoons of yoghurt on a sanitary towel and securing it in place in the usual way. Do not use a tampon because this carries its own potential risks. (If you have a period, switch to external protection, at least for the course of this disturbance.)

When not wearing the local application of yoghurt, try and let that area of the body breathe by avoiding tight-fitting synthetic underwear. Cotton panties are fine, and stockings are better than tights; best is not wearing any underwear at all. Try to avoid scented soaps and toiletries (adding half a cup of apple cider vinegar to the water each time you take a bath will help) and use plain white toilet tissue, making sure you wipe from front to back on every occasion.

Each night for three consecutive nights, insert a clove of garlic deep into the vagina as far as you can reach. For this to be effective you need to abstain from intercouse, but if the thrush is bad this will not be much of a problem. Peel a clove very carefully so as not to break the thin, inner layer of skin. Meanwhile, sterilise a sewing needle and thread it with a double thickness of sterilised sewing cotton. Thread the needle through the clove and tie it off. The thread will help you to remove the garlic in the morning, and it also allows a little of the potent garlic juice to seep out of the small hole that has been made, while ensuring that not enough escapes to irritate.

If the thrush has not cleared up after three days, discontinue the garlic insertion and douche twice daily with a dilution of apple cider vinegar instead. Douche kits are available from most chemists but there are two types. One type looks as though it is made to be carried around in a handbag and is so small as to be useless. You need a larger one that will allow large amounts of cleansing liquid to flush through the vagina.

Fill the douche container with warm water and add two tablespoons of apple cider vinegar for each 1.2 litres (2 pints) of water. Hang it on the shower rail or on a shelf in the bathroom. You will be using gravity as the only source of pressure for this, so the container needs to be placed above the level of the bath (do check that the tube is long enough to reach). Use the nozzle that has several small holes all around the top (some kits come with a choice of nozzles) and insert it very gently into the vagina whilst crouching down in the bath. Open the flow switch, or whatever contraption is used to regulate the flow of liquid and try to relax as it flows in and out of your body, cleansing as it goes. Some people like to lie down while this is going on, or you can stay crouched, but sitting down is not possible. Afterwards, take some time to relax, and don't worry if some of the douche fluid takes longer to come out.

If the thrush clears up quickly yet reappears regularly, consider following the three-day cleansing diet on page 20 and also think about consulting a naturopath or natural healthcare practitioner for some more personal advice. Women sometimes find that the symptoms reappear at a certain point in their cycle each month and this means that a more tailored health review is needed to produce the best results.

TONSILLITIS

Whatever you do, try and keep your tonsils. Although they may get swollen and inflamed on occasion, tonsils are on the front line of the body's defences and do a wonderful job.

Repeated attacks of tonsillitis show that the body's immune system could do with a boost. An improvement in your general diet, vitamin C up to saturation dose (see page 8), and large amounts of garlic each day will all help. Thyme will act here as a powerful antiseptic. If gargling is possible, do so with half a cup of cooled strong thyme tea and slowly sip the other half. Adding a few drops of essential oil of thyme to an oil burner will support this effect, and taking a facial sauna or steam bath with a drop or two of the oil added to the water will reinforce the mild local anaesthetic effect and help reduce the discomfort.

Mallow is another herb which has a soothing effect on the tonsils. Slowly sip two cups of hot mallow tea each day and enjoy the speedy relief it brings.

My favourite remedy is simply to gargle with red sage tea several times daily and to drink half a cup each day (see **Coughs and Sore Throats**). I have never known this to fail to bring relief. If it is reinforced with a hot compress on the throat, the sage can have a 'sandwich' effect on the tonsils, healing them from within and without. Steep two tablespoons of dried sage or a handful of fresh leaves in boiling water for about half a minute. Soak a piece of thin cotton fabric, long enough to wrap around your neck, in the liquid and wring it out. Wrap it around your throat and cover it immediately with a thick towel to help keep you dry and keep the heat in. Change this several times during the day and wear a cold compress at night. For a cold compress, soak a length of cotton fabric in cold water, wrap it around your throat and cover it with a towel. This is the most effective cure if the tonsils are very swollen and the neck is stiff and sore, but you must make sure the cotton fabric wraps around the neck in only one thickness – tea-towels are usually suitable for hydrotherapy measures but will be too wide in this case.

Another gargle that is very popular for its speedy results and pleasant taste is fenugreek. Make fenugreek tea by steeping two teaspoons of fenugreek seeds in a large mug of boiling water for about a minute. Strain the liquid and gargle with it when it has cooled sufficiently. This can be repeated up to four times a day.

TOOTHACHE

Just about all forms of toothache will respond to being packed with fresh propolis. This wonderful gift from bees sets tightly, making a better temporary filling than any manufactured material. Propolis has marked antibacterial properties and tastes rather good as well. It will keep in the fridge for ages and can also be frozen, so it is worth befriending your local beekeeper and purchasing a small amount. It has a myriad other uses and a piece the size of a match head can be taken regularly to support the immune system.

If propolis cannot be found, apply a little oil of clove (available from chemists) to the area by finger or on the tip of a cotton bud. If the tooth will allow, chew some raw cloves and the pain-killing effect will be doubled.

Dr Bach's Rescue Remedy applied to the tooth and dropped on to the skin outside the mouth at regular intervals will help, however acute the discomfort.

Using the joints of the fingers below the knuckles to apply pressure to the root of the teeth can have a wonderful pain-killing effect. The pressure needs to be applied for some minutes, or until the stinging pain stops. It is very easy to do; if you feel the area around your mouth you will find that the teeth seem to travel quite a long way into the surrounding bone. If the ache is in the upper teeth, you may need to push in just under your cheekbones to find the root, whereas for the lower teeth you need to press deeply into your chin. A drop of essential oil of sandalwood, diluted in a teaspoon or more of light oil such as soya, almond or pure unroasted sesame can be stroked on to the skin around the area you have worked on; this will provide further relief and also help heal any skin reaction.

There is currently a trend towards replacing amalgam dental fillings with white plastic. Both materials can be potentially hazardous and the greatest care needs to be taken when removing old amalgam fillings. It is worth discussing the procedures with your dentist weeks in advance if you intend to have this work done. Take the homoeopathic remedy amalgam 30 for a week before the dental work and the homoeopathic remedy arnica on the day and for three days afterwards. I also recommend that you take some naturally activated charcoal immediately before and after the appointment. Dr Bach's Rescue Remedy drops may help and can also be useful for anyone who is nervous about visiting their dentist.

To relieve any residual pain after a tooth has been extracted or lost, gently rub warmed olive oil into the outside of the face on the side where the tooth was. Then lie down on something soft and woolly to hold in the warmth.

ULCERS

Mouth ulcers are most often an early sign of a sluggish immune system, and it is advisable to heed their warning and treat the whole body as well as the site of the ulcers. Any of the measures for boosting your health will help (see pages 13–25). The most effective cure is to squeeze a few drops of juice from an organically grown fresh lemon directly on to the ulcer. It hurts, but only for a second, and if this can be repeated several times a day the ulcer will usually be gone within 24 hours. This cure also works for cold sores, which can accompany ulcers, particularly if the system is low.

Increase your vitamin C intake by eating at least one large mixed salad of raw vegetables each day. Vitamin C can be taken as a supplement with bioflavonoids; 1g a day with meals is the starting dose, rising gradually to 3g daily.

If recurrent mouth ulcers are a problem, it may be time to check your dental fillings. I have seen a number of mouth ulcers, cold sores and facial spots appear as a result of having amalgam fillings replaced. Unless this procedure is done with great care, you may experience reactions of this type for up to 18 months. Many dentists recommend taking a homoeopathic dose of amalgam 30 for one week prior to such work. A daily dose of 0.2ml echinacea tincture (if tolerated) plus a daily multi-vitamin and mineral supplement, is also advisable. (See also **Toothache**).

Ulcers on the body are best drawn to the attention of your

naturopath or natural healthcare practitioner. If they are troublesome, the gel from a fresh leaf of the aloe plant is particularly soothing and can be applied before going to bed. Try to leave the area uncovered throughout the day so it can breathe.

Alternatively, a combination of equal parts of dried comfrey root and slippery elm powder, mixed into a gel with coconut oil and secured with marshmallow leaves, makes a healing application. Again this can be applied at night and kept in place with a piece of cotton fabric, then removed in the morning so the skin is able to breathe during the day.

People troubled with stomach ulcers will find that there are many natural solutions and the best results will be gained through an individually tailored diet and healthcare plan from your naturopath or natural healthcare practitioner. In the meantime, short-term relief may be gained by drinking at least two cups each day of warm (not hot) slippery elm tea, and taking a glass of fresh cabbage juice up to five times a day. Both are very soothing, and will help normalise the stomach lining.

UPSET TUMMY

This often occurs when your system feels unsettled yet no specific ailments can be identified. There are a number of good home remedies to help settle the system but if aggravation continues, it is recommended that you seek the advice of your naturopath or natural healthcare practitioner.

Marshmallow flower tea is a wonderfully sweet and soothing drink that may be taken up to three times a day. It is best of all during the summer months when the flowers may be freshly picked and added straight to the pot. Brew for no more than two minutes, then sip the hot tea slowly. Fresh marshmallow flowers may also be added to salads and sandwiches; they taste delightful and bring a wonderful colour to meals along with their healing effects.

Swallowing three papaya seeds before each meal will help settle the tummy, and improve digestion of proteins if this is proving difficult. It is important to swallow them whole, not chew them. If you can skip a meal and eat the papaya instead, so much the better. A mixture of yoghurt and banana is another good meal substitute that is kind to the gut, filling and nutritious, and tastes delicious. Simply mix a carton of plain live goat's or sheep's milk yoghurt with two sliced bananas, or purée them together in a blender for a smooth consistency. One of my mother's standby remedies for settling a grumbling tummy is to take a tablespoon of sweet sherry in a small glass of warm milk. This always works well for her.

Bilberry extract, made by steeping freshly picked bilberries in brandy for three weeks, is an old folk remedy for keeping the gut working well. The drink is delicious, though, so I wonder whether the bilberry is to be praised, or the happiness it delivers.

Perhaps the most un-naturopathic remedy ever, one of the best cures for upset tummies is to drink a glass of slightly flat Coca-Cola. I'm not sure why this should work – something to do with the sugar-caffeine combination perhaps – but it settles upset tummy, nausea and even mild diarrhoea quite effectively. Do be sure, however, to brush your teeth well after drinking it.

URTICARIA

This is often called hives, or nettle rash, because the rash that covers the skin is similar to that caused by nettles. In this lies the cure, for nettles themselves are among the best treatments. Drinking several cups of fresh nettle tea every day and, if possible, also including the young nettle tops in a soup or broth each day, is one of the most cleansing and effective remedies. If fresh nettles are in short supply, one teaspoon of the bottled juice may be taken three times a day, or the tea may be made from dried nettles.

As with all skin complaints, treatment will focus on the diet, because this is one of the most effective ways of supporting the bowel – skin problems often indicate that the body's other eliminative routes are congested. Fasting and other constitutional work is best undertaken with the advice and support of your naturopath or natural healthcare practitioner. General dietary changes can make a huge difference, though, and avoiding sugars, saturated fats and fried food should quickly show an improvement.

A number of people develop urticaria as a reaction to a group of foods called salicylates. This group includes potatoes, cucumbers, peppers, tomatoes and some fruits – most berries and citrus fruits, grapes, cherries, apricots, apples, melons and plums. Almonds also contain a large amount of salicylic acid, and perhaps the biggest culprit is the food colouring tartrazine, sometimes called Yellow No. 5 or E102. This finds its way into a great many foodstuffs, so check labels carefully. A number of drugs contain salicylates too, the most common of which is aspirin.

Reducing the amount of salicylates in your diet may well decrease the incidence of this complaint. It's a good opportunity to increase the overall quality and freshness of the foods you eat, too. Try to increase vitamin and mineral levels by having at least one large, mixed raw salad every day, plus three additional servings of fresh fruit or vegetables. This will help on a constitutional level and assist the body in its battle against stress.

Stress can be divided into two types, both of which have a marked effect on health. External stress is something we are all familiar with: work pressures, money worries, family concerns – anything that originates outside ourselves and makes us feel below par. The body's response is to rise to meet the challenge, and this can be very depleting to energy reserves. Internal stress can be caused by too much external stress – having to function while deeply weary from too much pressure – and also by a number of natural internal mechanisms, such as continued immune function and general metabolism. Increased internal stress may well be responsible for the heightened histamine reaction resulting in the rash-like spread of weals or blisters that characterises urticaria. This means that anything you can do to improve your general health and reduce stress levels will have a direct effect upon the hives.

The essential oils of chamomile and melissa both work on the underlying causes of allergic responses, as well as being specifically aimed at skin function. Their calming qualities can be most useful here. Both oils may be placed in an oil burner and two drops of each can be added to a warm bath. If the affected area of skin is small enough, add two drops of each essential oil to 300ml (½ pint) of warm water and sponge it on directly. This is useful if itchiness is severe.

If you have large weals, applying a fresh cabbage leaf will give some relief. Rinse a leaf well in cold water and apply it straight to the affected site. You can keep it in place by tying a large piece of cotton cloth over it. For larger areas, take some of the biggest external cabbage leaves and cover them with boiling water for a few seconds until you can crush the tough central stem. Then plunge them into cold water and apply to the skin.

To treat the whole body, take an oatmeal bath (see **Eczema**). Stay in the bath for as long as you like – in warmer weather it may be pleasant to remain in the bath for longer periods while the water cools and becomes even more refreshing. Heat generally aggravates urticaria, while coolness always seems to improve it.

VARICOSE VEINS

These most often appear in the legs and can result from poor circulation or from periods of increased abdominal pressure arising from pregnancy, obesity, persistent constipation, etc. The swollen, stretched veins can be the source of much irritation and discomfort, causing swelling and distension of the whole area and making walking and other exercise difficult. Varicose veins can appear in any other area, including the abdomen and the breasts.

I have heard of cases of varicose veins being caused by negligent leg waxing. This method of hair removal must be used with great care. If the wax is too hot, the skin tender or the removal haphazard, considerable damage may be done to the delicate peripheral veins in the area.

Rutin is a good supplement to take if these veins are a problem, and localised applications of cooling witch hazel can help enormously. Keep the clearly marked bottle in the fridge and apply it to the affected area twice a day with cotton wool. Taking 1–2g of vitamin C each day and 200–400iu of vitamin E will help improve the circulation and build the collagen needed for healthy vein walls.

If the legs are affected, keeping them raised above the level of your heart for at least 20 minutes each day can have a dramatically beneficial long-term effect. This is easiest in bed but can be done anywhere or at any time – while you watch television, read a book, massage your tummy, or do any number of things. It is also a good idea to raise the foot of your bed by about 10cm (4 inches) – easily done by placing a few old telephone directories or similar underneath the legs.

Try to avoid standing still for long periods of time or, if this is impossible, shift the weight from one foot to another or rest one foot on a small stool. When sitting, avoid crossing the legs, and try to exercise the area to strengthen it and tone the muscles. Cycling or stationary cycling are among the best specific exercises for varicose veins in the legs.

Regular weight-bearing exercise such as walking, particularly barefoot in the early-morning dew, or cold-water paddling, will help tone the legs, and hot sage tea compresses will give enormous relief. Make a pot of strong sage tea and, when it is cool enough to touch, soak a cotton handkerchief or thin cotton tea-towel in the liquid, wring it out and apply to the affected area. Repeat once it has cooled. This can be done several times each day and is very quick acting.

See also **Constipation** and **Poor Circulation**.

VOMITING

This is one of the fastest and most effective ways for the body to expel toxic material so it is often best to allow it to continue and then treat the person and help them settle. In the case of children, and where projectile vomiting occurs, then medical attention should be sought.

If the vomited matter has been particularly bitter and foul-tasting, lie down and placing a Swedish bitters compress directly on the stomach to settle the system and soothe away any remaining distress. First cover the skin with a thin dressing of calendula cream or unroasted sesame oil. Apply several drops of the Swedish bitters to a piece of thin cotton fabric (a handkerchief is ideal) dampened with a little cold water and then place it on the left side of the chest immediately below the nipple and extending down towards the waist. Leave in place until the compress has dried and any nausea has disappeared.

For more fatty substances, wash the mouth out with a dill infusion. Take large amounts of fresh dill and cram it into a teapot. Fill with boiling water and leave to stand for about three minutes, then strain and allow to cool. If the fresh herb cannot be found, two teaspoons of dried dill may be used instead. Wash the mouth out with the infusion and then slowly sip a cupful to which has been added a pinch of cloves. This should soon settle the stomach and have a pleasant, calming effect on the whole person.

Vomiting is a drastic thing for the body to do and afterwards the sufferer needs to be 'wrapped in cotton wool' and receive lots of rest and gentle care for the following 48 hours. A very simple diet, regular cups of liquorice root tea, warm baths – and even candlelight and sweet music! – are all prescribed.

Walking barefoot on the earth is a wonderful way of settling the body after an upset like this. Any patch of clean ground will suffice – my own favourite is tallish grass, so that with each step the foot seems to disappear into a lush green carpet. Sitting on the earth is also deeply settling, particularly if you lean back against a tree trunk. You may be able to feel the strength and support of the tree behind you as you are cradled and nourished by the earth herself. Even if you are not aware of these feelings, the occasion is no less healing, so just relax and enjoy.

WARTS AND VERUCCAE

These small, often hard growths in the outer layer of the skin are thought to be caused by a virus, and may be very persistent. Warts can appear anywhere on the body, although the hands, neck and genitals are the most common sites, while veruccae are confined to the feet. They can spread quite easily once they have taken hold and it is a sensible precaution to protect others by, for example, not having unprotected sex if genital warts are present, and wearing flip-flops or similar shoes in swimming pool areas if you have veruccae.

The best natural cure I know is to rub the affected area with a freshly cut piece of organically grown lemon as many times a day as possible. It may be the local application of vitamin C that does the trick, but I feel that there is real magic to be found in lemons and I use them to help with all sorts of conditions, including warts, ulcers and dry skin.

More stubborn warts and verrucae may respond to repeated applications of two drops of tea-tree or ti-tree essential oil diluted in a tablespoon of water or oil. A neat application of tincture of homoeopathic thuja left to dry in the sun may be dramatically effective. However, thuja should not be taken internally or applied externally for longer than one month without the monitoring of your naturopath or natural healthcare practitioner.

Warts have a very bad press and people often regard them as negative, unsightly 'hate spots'. Dr Bach's Crab Apple is a good remedy to take three times daily if such negative personal feelings are a part of the difficulty. It can also be applied directly to the warts and the surrounding area.

SUPPLIERS, CENTRES AND USEFUL ADDRESSES

The following addresses are not intended as a comprehensive list, nor is inclusion necessarily an endorsement.

Ayurved Health Centres:

Dr Naram's Ayurveda International Ltd
220 Andrew's Building
Queen Street
Cardiff CF1 4AU
Tel: 01222 238467

Maharishi Ayurved Health Centres:

The Golden Dome
Woodley Park
Skelmersdale
Lancashire WN8 6UQ
Tel: 01695 51008

2112F Street NW Suite 503
Washington DC 20037
USA
Tel: 001 (202) 785 2700

32 2nd Avenue
St Peters
South Australia 5069
Australia
Tel: 00 61(8) 362 8336

National Centre
5 Adam Street
Greenlane
Auckland 5
New Zealand
Tel: 00 64(9) 9592 252599 619

Suppliers of Hopi Ear Candles:

BioSun
Sheepcoates Lane
Great Totham
Maldon
Essex CM9 8NT

Eryri Trading Post
Hafod Ysbyty
Cwm Teigl
Llan ffestiniog
Gwynedd LL41 4RF

Twin Light Trails
PO Box 52
London N10 3TQ

Twin Light Trails
11024 Montgomery NE
Suite 166
Albuquerque
New Mexico 87111-3962
USA

Cranial Work:

Cranio-Sacral Therapy Association of the UK
3 Sandygrove Cottages
Horsley
Nailsworth
Gloucestershire GL6 0PS

Karuna Core Therapies
Curtisknowle House
Curtisknowle
near Totnes
Devon TQ7 7JX
Tel: 0154 882 583

The Cranial Academy
Meridian
Idaho 83642
USA

Naturopathic Associations:

Incorporated Society of British Naturopaths
Kingston
The Coach House
293 Gilmerton Road
Edinburgh EH16 5UQ
Tel: 0131 664 3435

Incorporated Society of Registered Naturopaths
1 Albermarle Road
The Mount
York YO2 1EN

United Osteopathic Physician's Guild Ltd
112 Essillia Street
Collaroy Plateau
New South Wales 2097
Australia
Tel: 00 61(2) 981 4319

Chi Dynamics:

Centre for Harmony
PO Box 109
Gloucester
Gloucestershire GL2 9YD
Tel: 01452 382 536

Natural Health Spas:

Bartragh Centre
Bartragh Island
Lillala Bay
County Mayo
Eire
Tel: (353 96) 32285

Cloona Health Centre
Westport
County Mayo
Eire
Tel: (353 98) 25251

Tyringham Naturopathic Clinic,
Newport Pagnall
Buckinghamshire
MK16 9ER
Tel: 0190 8610450

Dr Bach's Flower Remedies:

The Edward Bach Centre
Mount Vernon
Sotwell
Wallingford
Oxon OX10 0PZ
Tel: 01491 39489

Flower Essence Society (flowers from outside the UK)
PO Box 459
Nevada City
California 95959
USA
Tel: 00 1 (800) 548 0075

General Suppliers:

G. Baldwin and Co, Herbs
171/173 Walworth Road
London SE17 1RW
Tel: 0171 703 5550

John Bell and Croyden
52–54 Wigmore Street
London W1H 9DG
Tel: 0171 935 5555

Gerard House
3 Wickham Road
Boscombe
Bournemouth
Dorset BH7 6JX
Tel: 01202 434116

Green Farm Nutrition Centre
Burwash Common
East Sussex TN19 7LX
Tel: 01435 382482

The Herb Society
PO Box 599
London SW11 4RW
Tel: 0171 823 5583

The Herbal Apothecary
103 High Street
Syston
Leicester LE7 8GQ
Tel: 01162 602690

Lambert's Nutritional Suppliers
1 Lambert's Road
Tunbridge Wells
Kent TN2 3EQ
Tel: 01892 513116

Lanes Health Products
Sisson Road
Gloucester GL1 3QB

Micheline Arcier Aromatherapy
7 William Street
London SW1X 9HL
Tel: 0171 235 3545

Natural Touch Ltd
Organic Essential Oils
29 Gordondale Road
Wimbledon
London SW19 8EN
Tel: 0181 944 8437

Neal's Yard Apothecary
15 Neal's Yard
London WC2H 9DP
Tel: 0171 379 7222

New World Cassettes
16a Neal's Yard
London WC2H 9DP
Tel: 0171 379 5972

Potters Ltd
Leyland Mill Lane
Wigan
Lancashire WN1 2SB

Verde Essential Oils
75 Northcote Road
London SW11
Tel: 0171 924 4379

Weleda (UK) Ltd
Heanor Road
Ilkeston
Derbyshire
Tel: 01602 303151

Wholistic Research Company
Bright Haven
Robin's Land
Lolworth
Cambridge CB3 8HH
Tel: 01954 781074

Other Useful Addresses:

Compassion in World Farming
20 Lavant Street
Petersfield
Hampshire GU32 3EW
Tel: 01730 64208

Council for Complementary and Alternative Medicine
179 Gloucester Place
London NW1 6DX
Tel: 0171 724 9103

Humane Slaughter Association
(Council of Justice to Animals)
34 Blanche Lane
South Mimms
Potters Bar
Hertfordshire EN6 3PA
Tel: 01707 59040

Institute for Complementary Medicine
Unit 4
Tavern Quay
Rope Street
Rotherhithe
London SE16 1AA
Tel: 0171 636 9543

The Soil Association
86 Colston Street
Bristol BS1 5BB
Tel: 01179 290661

FURTHER READING

An A–Z of Natural Healthcare, Belinda Grant (Optima 1993)

Acupressure – *How to Cure Common Ailments the Natural Way*, Michael Reed Gach (Piatkus, 1990)

Aromatherapy, An A–Z, Patricia Davis (C.W. Daniel Co 1991)

As I See It, Betty Balcombe (Piatkus, 1994)

Better Health through Natural Healing, Ross Trattler, ND DO (Thorsons, 1984)

Chinese Medicine – The Web That Has No Weaver, Ted J Kaptcuk (Rider Books, 1983)

The Detox Diet Book, Belinda Grant (Optima, 1991)

The Energy Connection, Betty Balcombe (Piatkus, 1993)

Food Combining for Health, Doris Grant and Jean Joice (Thorsons, 1984)

Food For Free, Richard Mabey (Fontana Press, 1972)

A Guide to Biochemic Tissue Salts, Dr Andrew Stanway (Van Dyke Books, 1982)

A Guide to the Bach Flower Remedies, Julian Barnard (C.W. Daniel Co, 1986)

Joy's Way, W. Brugh Joy MD (J. P. Archer, Inc, 1979)

Kitty Campion's Handbook of Herbal Health, Kitty Campion (Sphere Books, 1985)

The Medicine Way, Kenneth Meadows (Element, 1990)

Nature through the Seasons, Richard Adams and Max Hooper (Penguin, 1975)

Perfect Health, Deepak Chopra, MD (Bantam, 1990)

The Way of the Shaman, Michael Harner (Harper Collins, 1980)

INDEX